NEUROPLASTICITY

Simple Strategies to Better Manage Your Life

(How to Boost Neurogenesis and Rewire Your
Brain With Light)

Susan Smith

Published By John Kembrey

Susan Smith

All Rights Reserved

Neuroplasticity: Simple Strategies to Better Manage Your Life (How to Boost Neurogenesis and Rewire Your Brain With Light)

ISBN 978-1-77485-252-1

Legal & Disclaimer

Table of Contents

Introduction

How is it that brain plasticity becomes crucial? Because you are able to literally alter the brain's wiring. The brain is built to be able to change. This is the way it was designed to help you survive. Your brain is designed to feel comfortable. It doesn't want to be uncomfortable. That's why psychologists claim that around 95% of your daily life will be run by the subconscious. We have approximately 65,000 thoughts per every day. Between 75 and 90% of these thoughts come from your default brain. They're on autopilot in a sense. This is great if you've cultivated your neural pathways and trained your mind to think positive. We must break free from the way we've been programmed to think. thinking. Our surroundings, our conditions and those we spend the majority of our time with , and their habits and beliefs (which they've acquired) influence and shape our minds. The majority of our beliefs are only derived from those who have the closest relationship with. You're who you are with. You won't be flying with Eagles if you hang around with turkeys. You've probably heard those statements before. It's even Proverbs 13:20 teaches us that those who follow wise men will be wiser, however those who are fools will be afflicted. Your circumstances in life and what you think is the fault of you because you've been living in the default mode. You've been through the routines day in and out, based on what you've discovered, observed, and witnessed so far. Today is a brand new day! It's no longer necessary to remain in default mode.

What is the influence that has shaped your opinions?

This is a critical issue to consider. Why do you believe and accept what you believe? As a child, each when my mom introduced me to someone unfamiliar she would inform them that I was shy and had didn't have confidence in myself. I was told that repeatedly over and over and over. The idea was embedded in my brain. I'm certain that my mother did not intend to hurt anyone. She's an amazing person. Perhaps she believed she was trying to help me in some way, by explaining my scared behavior at one point or another and it then was the standard. It was a way of life. It was ingrained in her brain. My grandmother passed away in the early years of my mother's life. She was young. Her father was an alcohol addict and a slap-daddy to nearly all of the family members. My mother recalls feeling as like she wasn't valued or felt loved. My mother told me that she always said that if she had kids she would do all she could to ensure they felt loved and wanted. She was as good as she could and was intentional in at the very least showing us how much we loved. While she was unaware she was rewiring the brain of her in a positive way. She broke through the learned behaviour of abuse as well. My mother was extremely poor in her childhood and the poverty mindset was taught and, over time, was embedded in her brain. As a result we were constantly told that there was not enough money, that money doesn't grow on trees or the fact that "we couldn't afford it". This skewed thinking was ingrained to my mind as real-world reality and despite working to the max but I didn't have enough funds. I worked several jobs at once and yet I was unable to save a dime. It was a belief I had learned that was ingrained into my brain via repetition.

Do you know anyone who criticizes a lot often? In which criticism is their primary concern? In which you are unable to be sure of your actions? People who are critical are hard to get along with. They are often unable to giving compliments to others. They are known to complain frequently. They love to talk about other people. Don't be too difficult on them. The brains of these people have been programmed to function this way over the course of time. They had a critical day the first day, next day, and the next day, and without conscious of it, they rewired their brains to function to react, react and think in this manner. The neural pathways they have created are so powerful in this field, that it's now an integral element of their identity. It is now their default brain. It's automatic. The only way to change is to be aware of the issue and to take action to reverse all that was accomplished. It's a long process and requires a lot of effort however, it is possible to get it accomplished. Critical thinking is not an appropriate characteristic to possess. If someone who is critical wants to change their behavior the only thing they need to do is work to create new neural pathways that lead to being positive and optimistic. They can also be supportive. This requires a small amount of work but less than. When we begin to move moving in a different direction is the moment that neural pathways begin to develop. Utilize it or let it go. If we stop being critical by noticing these moments and then immediately changing the thought, the neural pathways that surround criticism will begin to diminish and eventually disintegrate.

The brain is built to change. It is possible to alter your brain to make it better or for worse. If you concentrate on the negatives it can strengthen the neuronal pathways within your brain. It will make negativity a prominent feature and an integral element of your life. Negativity will become a default behavior for you. If you are focused on finding the positive in all situations, you'll be creating building neural pathways and strengthening them towards being positive. This becomes a aspect of your daily life. The best part is that we have the power to pick and choose. We don't have to allow random thoughts dictate our lives. It is no longer necessary to be in an unfavorable default mode. Doubt, worry, judgements and opinions, lack of thinking or bad habits and more. can be changed and become are now a thing of the past.

How effective you wish to be, no matter how successful you want to be or however big your ambitions ultimately down to the sequence of your actions and reactions which you both consciously and subconsciously manage. Every action you take is echoed into the future, becoming the story of tomorrow. Your actions that shape your current state result directly from your mental state. Your mind is built upon the brain's faculties that are built on the brain's physical structure.

Although this book isn't meant to be used as an instruction in neuropsychology, it's goal is to guide the reader to become familiar with the language, nomenclature and the functioning of the brain's underpinnings as well as to understand the concept of brain and the way it connects to beliefs, thoughts or mindsets, and the actions they take. What's about to be described in this book is a bit simplified and is designed to meet the reader in the same place and does not presume any knowledge of neuroscience or psychology.

The chapters start with the brain's physical structure and consider it to be an organ that is only that, not much more. It is an essential base for understanding the mind that is a part on top of the brain. We are careful to explain that the mind isn't the brain, and the reverse is true. A tangible object is perceivable through touch and sight. However the mind is not able to have tangible nature and is purely intangible.

The combination of these various mentalities results in different characters people can create throughout their lives. Three elements make up the person who impacts and influences the world surrounding them. The first one is the experience that the individual was exposed to as well as the beliefs taught to the person and the third is the impact of compounding.

Once we have a better understanding of the brain and the complexities it has to offer and its functions, we are in a position to begin to understand the concept of neuroplasticity. The name itself implies the fact that your brain (the part that is the neuro in the word) is malleable , like plastic. It has a degree of flexibility and the ability to adapt and change (the plasticity component in the term medical.)

The brain is divided into two distinct parts. The primitive brain, which is concerned with the fundamental living conditions and the more advanced brain which produces more advanced thinking and actions. Each is influenced by the other, and this influence manifests itself in various ways.

The brain is adaptable and you are able to change it by yourself! You're capable of rewiring the brain, and anyone is able to accomplish it! The brain can be reprogrammed. Are you excited by this latest discovery? You should be thrilled!

The brain is built to change. It is possible to change or rewire the brain regardless. Why not take your time? If you can truly comprehend the dynamics that are taking place the brain, you will be able to make better decisions for yourself. If you focus and notice on negative events, typically you create the neural connections in your brain. This can allow negativity to become a normal element of your life. Negativity is the default setting for you. If you are focused on finding the positive in every circumstance, you will create and form neural pathways that promote positive thinking and this will be your default mode. You can pick. We don't need to let random thoughts and opinions, as well as opinions of other people, that are ingrained subconsciously in our brains, dictate our lifestyle.

It is possible to find that some of the things have been mentioned throughout the book. There aren't many, just some key details. This is intentional since repetition is among the key factors to developing your neuropathways. If you feel that you're bored by certain scientific aspects that are in this book you can simply go through the book and then shift to what is most appealing to you.

I have witnessed a number of successes and positive changes occur for my clients when they began practicing and applying the knowledge they'd learned. The brain can be rewired to benefit you in most incredible ways. Let's get started! Your incredible, happy and healthy, fulfilling prosperous, successful life is waiting for you!

Chapter 1: How Brain Plasticity Can Benefit You

The most up-to-date and most recent brain research inform us our brains are more flexible and flexible than we originally believed. If you think of the brain being hard and rigid it is not. Indeed all through our lives we are able to shape our brains, develop, and enhance our cognitive capabilities and our intelligence level. What's amazing to know is this dispels the idea that we can not do anything to make up for the missed opportunities to improve our intelligence as we grew older. We can take a great deal of steps to develop our brains , no matter age.

There are two methods to reap the benefits of this. The first is to understand the mechanisms and brain's dynamics by learning to fully control it. The other alternative is to find new ways to improve the abilities you already have. One of the most important aspects is achieving the right equilibrium between EQ (emotional quality) as well as your IQ (intelligence quote). A key component of brain development is raising your awareness of the way your brain actually functions.

To fully comprehend the idea of brain plasticity, you must first comprehend the current view of intelligence. In the new view developed by Howard Gardner, it was believed that intelligence is available in a variety of types. This differs from the conventional notion that intelligence can be assessed through observing the capabilities of a person's brain. Based on the concept that there are multiple levels of intelligence, the brain could be described as a complete and multi-purpose machine. It functions independently of content and context.

Howard Gardner, tagged as the founder of many intelligences believed that there are eight distinct kinds of intelligence. This is an astonishment to the common belief that intelligence can be evaluated by examining verbal, analytical, and mathematical capabilities. Are you aware that over the passage of time, more and more millionaires made by our society aren't possessing any university degrees? This is a clear proof that college may be successful in fostering certain types of intelligence, but not all.

By mastering the art of brain plasticity, you'll discover how to enhance not only your cognitive capabilities. Additionally, you will have the opportunity to develop other areas of intelligence. You may be wondering which capabilities can be developed by the strategies that are prescribed to you by the brain's plasticity. These are the various intelligences as per Howard Gardner:

Verbal-linguistic is the ability of a person to effectively use words and recognize linguistic phrases immediately. The people who are poets, speakers and teachers possess this ability, and can communicate their ideas through written and spoken words.

Logical-mathematical: This intelligence applies to engineers, accountants, and scientists. It's the ability to apply principles of logic and the rules of math. This is evident in the ability to solve mathematical and scientific difficulties easily. These have the ability to be "naturals" when they are working with numbers. They are able to easily discern patterns and connections.

Visual-spatial: Sculptors and architects, visual artists and pilots are superior in this area. They are conscious of spatial relationships of objects. They are also adept at visualizing, particularly when it comes to perspectives. The people with the most advanced visual-spatial ability can effortlessly manipulate the mental image of objects, draw out existing patterns, alter the scope of vision and recognize the relative dimensions.

Body-kinesthetic: They are the most aware of their sensations and movements. They also have excellent hand-eye coordination. They excel in controlling fluid and physical movements. They retain information by doing, and also use their muscles to store information. The most notable examples of people who are highly skilled in this area include athletes, mechanics surgeons, dancers, and mechanics.

Interpersonal: CEOs, Leaders and politicians, pastors and psychologists are generally superior in this area. This is because they are able to be able to react and recognize signals that cannot be communicated by words. They are able to see the world through others' eyes. They excel in their interactions with other people. They are able to discern people's thoughts, feelings and motives.

Musical: DJs, conductors and songwriters are recognized for their natural ease and tuned to music, sound and rhythm. They are also able to pinpoint the pitch of voice, tunes, and tonality. They are able to compose music, perform or simply enjoy the art.

Intrapersonal These are those who are adept at the inner workings of their own thoughts and emotions. They are able to interpret their own moods, attitudes and physical signals. They are seeking to gain a better understanding of their personal motives, feelings desire, motivations, and feelings. It is evident in individuals such as spiritual leaders entrepreneurs, artists, and spiritual leaders.

Natural: They're sensitive to nature's elements and world. They are interested in the natural surroundings and the animals that inhabit it. This is best demonstrated by botanists, geologists and biologists.

For the record, the brain functions like a young puppy. It can be taught. It is just a matter of having be able to "befriend" your own so that you are at ease teaching it new techniques. There are many techniques you could employ and you can find out the details about these techniques in this guide.

Chapter 2: Not So Fast

The same characteristics of neuroplasticity which make your brain more resilient makes it more vulnerable to external or internally (usually subconscious) adverse influences. If you live in a stressful environment and a poor upbringing or genetic mental illnesses, neuroplasticity could result in depressive, over-reactive or obsessive, anxious, and depressive patterns.

The Science of Neuroplasticity

So, what's going on behind the curtain about the brain's resilience? We'll provide an easy explanation of what's happening in your brain whenever it undergoes changes. Being aware of what's going on in your mind is the initial step towards taking positive steps that produce positive results. It is important to be enthusiastic about this. You can live the life you want! It's yours to have and you've got a brain designed to lead you to where you want to go.

Your brain is comprised of 100 billion or more neurons which form approximately 10,000 connections with other neurons. (These connection points are referred to as synapses). Keep in mind this section about connecting neurons - this bit of information is crucial to understand the workings of neuroplasticity.

We're talking about an event in which neuronal synapses (connections) and pathways are altered due to behavioral as well as environmental and, finally the neural processes.

Fun Facts About Neurons

Neurons communicate with each other through chemical signals that travel through the synapse (the connection between neurons)

Neuronal impulses are an essential aspect of the way that the brain works . Neural impulses are the code that codes your thoughts, actions, and even your experiences.

The thoughts, actions and experiences alter your brain's structure as well as function. neural pathways which neurons use to talk to one another. This allows the brain to be responsive to everything around it.

Release of neurotransmitters is also influenced by the patterns of neural impulses.

A neurotransmitter chemical is released by a nerve cell. The chemical sends an information from a nerve cells to another, or to the muscle, organ or tissue.

A neurotransmitter is the transmission of a signal from one cell to the next.

Amazing stuff, right? Here's an example of this: Neurons transmit signals across connections. They result in the thought. The thought alters the way your neurons communicate with each other, which means that you are able to react in a way that is appropriate. If you are having an unfavorable thought then a neurotransmitter will be released from a nerve cells, sending a message to muscles of your face, instructing them to smile.

Are you confused? Don't worryabout it, by the time you finish this book, you'll be an expert in the inner functioning of neuroplasticity.

Chapter 3: Applications Of

Neuroplasticity

The brain can be described as a powerful organ that can store massive quantities of information and process it. Neuroplasticity has led to a variety of applications used by diverse medical disciplines. This chapter will talk about the various applications of neuroplasticity.

Treating Brain Damage

A variety of studies show that brain plasticity could aid in the recovery of the brain after any type of injury. Many neurologists utilize brain plasticity within the context of rehabilitating the brain. it is crucial to note that the mature brain isn't connected to a single neural circuit. There are numerous wirings within the brain that develop as a result of injuries. Contrary to what the majority of people believe the neural connections do not actually die with age. There is evidence from science that the cortical as subcortical rewiring of our brains is a response to injury or training. There is growing evidence to suggest of neurons (the process of generating the brain's new cells) can occur also in mammalian adult brains.

In a study conducted in 2006by researchers, they were working with patients suffering from strokes, which are characterized by the impediment of blood flow to the brain, thereby affecting the patient's movement. The research revealed that brain injuries triggered the process of reorganization on the brain. There is a chance of using brain plasticity when treating stroke patients.

The most straightforward way to think of neuroplasticity as a method of treating brain damage is to see it as a method to be able to learn again. Keep in mind that through your life, the brain relies on the fundamental neurobiological processes to acquire behavior or memories, as well as experiences. So, even after a brain injury there are left-over neural circuits that can modify and encode new behavior. Here are the changes that occur following the brain injury is sustained after the patient is subjected to training in brain plasticity.

Synapses undergo more changes like synaptogenesis. As a result, the neurons are more likely to lengthen and grow multiple projections to make stronger neural connections.

Studies also show an increase in neuron growth in specific regions in the hippocampus, dentate gyrus and the subventricular zone.

Angiogenesis can also be stimulated when people do neuroplasticity exercise. It is the process in which new blood vessels are created from damaged blood vessels that were already present. The availability of blood vessels to the brain is essential since the brain requires Oxygen.

Brains also experience fluctuations in excitability. This is a sign of the capacity of neurons to produce action potentials, which produce electric signals , which result in being able to fire with a high frequency of synapses.

Brain training improves the structure of neural networks through the growth of axons and cortical structures and the recruitment of brain cells.

Improvement of Vision

Brain training is also believed as a way to reverse decline in vision caused by age. Many doctors are now using an eye system training program for the brain in order to enable the brain to correct for any blurred image that is captured through the eye.

The ability of the visual system to the system of visual perception in your brain to alter its numerous responses to different variations that occur in visual information. Studies have shown that practice with various visual tasks is proven to boost performance and sensitivity of the eyes to specific vision. When we engage in visual activities the photoreceptors of the retina are altered which results in increased sensitivity and performance as a result of stimulation. This could lead to the elimination of various vision disorders like lazy eye.

As we get older, the eyes begin to see fuzzy images in the brain in a greater way than they did prior to. When the brain begins receiving more blurry information from your eyes as well as the detail that are displayed appear to be having less contrast in comparison to the reality. For instance, as the decrease in near vision, the sensitivity to initial contrast is less than the norm.

When you do brain plasticity, you're causing the neurons in the eye system process images at a low contrast, believing that this is the most efficient capability for the brain. The use of brain plasticity for treating vision issues encourages interconnection between neurons and neurons of the brain.

Learning Difficulties

Individuals with dyslexia or other learning disabilities may benefit from the process of brain plasticity. A study was conducted with those suffering from cognitive decline (ARCD) Patients must complete six exercises specifically designed to correct the problems in cognition, memory and motor control. Participants who exercised for between 8 and 10 weeks saw significant improvements on their ability. However, those with autism or attention deficit disorder could benefit from exercises for brain plasticity to enhance their abilities to learn. Here are some types of learning issues which can be addressed by using neuroplasticity exercises.

Dyslexia: Dyslexia is a kind of reading disorder which is characterized by difficulty understanding sounds, letters and words that rhyme. Children suffering from this condition suffer delays in their language development as they get older.

Dysgraphia: Dysgraphia is characterized by having incorrect and distorted handwriting. In addition to affecting your brain's function, the condition comes from issues with fine motor abilities. Apart from having problems in writing, people suffering from dysgraphia may also have difficulty to zip their jackets or tie shoelaces.

Dyspraxia: Dyspraxia is a disorder in which tasks that require fine motor control as well as balance and kinesthetic coordination are challenging, and those who suffer from this disorder are termed unsteady. They also show delayed speech.

Dyscalculia The disorder is caused by problems with learning that usually involve numerical abilities. The people suffering from this disorder are unable to comprehend complex math concepts and basic ones.

Chronic Pain

Patients who experience chronic pain from injury may benefit from neuroplasticity. In the course of tissue injury and inflammation, harmful stimuli can trigger different reactions to the nervous system's central nerve, which can, in turn, stimulate neuroplastic responses on the cortical level in order to alter the structure of the area that is affected and resulting in central sensitization.

A study conducted on patients with chronic regional pain syndrome, it was found that there was a decreases in their cortical Somatotopic representation, as well as the size of grey matter, thereby increasing the neural connections as well as increasing the desensitization of their affected region. Brain plasticity can be utilized to treat various chronic pain disorders, such as carpal tunnel syndrome, and low back pain that is chronic.

The causes of chronic pain are not discovered by researchers. However, one thing is certain and that is that people suffering with chronic pain could benefit from exercises that stimulate the brain. When individuals engage in activities such as exercise for motor skills, the performance increases due to the neuroplastic changes within their brain.

Researchers at The Brigham and Women's Hospital in Boston discovered that a particular network of brain areas known as"the Default Mode Network results to changes in the neural connections. The research indicates that changes in brain's connectivity indicate a general aspect of chronic pain. Therefore, it is essential to perform exercises to regulate the neural connections related to pain.

Chapter 4: No Longer A Concept, But

A Fact Of Life

Neuroplasticity is the natural capacity for the brain adapt and reorganize itself due to experience and learning. When you are struck by a thought and you think about it, your brain makes an synapse (the structure that allows neurons to send electrical or chemical messages to another nerve) to convey the thought. When you are learning new information the brain's new neurons (neurons) are developed to store this information as memories. When you sleep the brain constructs the new neural bridges (new synapses) and removes older bridges (old synapses). These are the primary manifestations of neuroplasticity in action.

The brain is always busy by creating new connections and cutting existing connections. It's constantly evolving in function and shape as new connections are made between neurons due to stimuli triggered by experience or learning. It is always occupied with the ongoing process of re-modelling existing synapses by altering and strengthening, stabilizing and pruning them to achieve an optimal level of functioning and provide a suitable response to each stimulation throughout the day. It may even alter the function of specific neurons when the situation calls for it, or re-route tasks through the creation of new neural pathways in the event of damage to brain cells. All of these are neural plasticity processes that keep our brain active all the time even when we're asleep.

The brain can handle multi-neuroplasticity processes such as those in a variety of locations simultaneously. If you're wondering how the brain can control these processes (which include billions of neurons connected to one another by millions of synapses) simultaneously all at once it is due to the extensive multi sensory integration of neurons within the human brain, allowing them to work as a single network to accomplish tasks in reaction to a stimulus or something that has affected the brain's actions. The triggers are what that cause the brain to trigger the neurons into the action. These triggers could come from a single word to an experience, a memory or an experience, learning, the surroundings, and everything else that can affect the brain.

To gain a deeper understanding of the triggers that cause changes in neurons' behavior it is necessary to look down to the neurons and observe what happens there. What we'll see is a tiny, tiny neuron which can house a massive an axon (the protoplasmic projection that originates from an cellular body that connects to another neuron , and is cells' signal transmission). The axon may spread from the spinal cord all the way to the foot, and connect 10,000 dendrites (a similar protoplasmic projection, which serves as a signals receiver) to create synapses.

Neurons are hungry for knowledge and are always seeking them. When they encounter new information or triggers, the neurons could begin to form connections with other neurons quickly. They could also simply strengthen their existing bonds to other neurons by making more synapses between their Axons. (This is usually what happens when we grow older, as when we reach that age, we've already got sufficient of the crucial neural connections we require in their place.) In addition to generating neurons and creating synapses in the brain, it also reduces the neural networks it has by removing synapses that have not been used in a long time or not utilized at all. The entire process is referred to as synaptic pruning. It is an ongoing brain activity in which synaptic connections are either removed or rebuilt based on their usage.

Synaptic pruning is a vital procedure that ensures that the brain doesn't spend its precious resources on the neural network that is of no or no value at all. This is the same procedure employed to eliminate defective or injured neural networks. Be aware that we were conceived with more synapses and neuronal cells than we'll ever require in our adult lives. The removal of synaptic connections rarely used is the brain's method of ensuring its efficiency.

There are instances that are not used, but crucial abilities are also cut. This may be the cause for the frequent forgetfulness or memory loss that which we frequently experience as we get older. It's also why the brain can be described as an 'use it or lose organ. Memory lapses could be due to the deterioration of neural connections as a result of the loss of frequently utilized synapses (synaptic pruning).

Our capacity to remember memory, recall abilities, or acquire new skills depends in synaptic pruning. We are more likely to succeed in tasks with many neural connections, especially when these connections are solid.

The knowledge we have gained can be used to make use of neuroplasticity to be more effective in accomplishing a specific task. When we are aware of the task that we are performing and continually doing the task at hand and allowing the neurons to generate more synapses and build neural connections that are specific to the task at hand. Be aware that only thought triggers the brain to act. The many and strengthened neuronal connections can make it simpler for us to complete the task, and perhaps even succeed in it. Not less than Aristotle mentioned this many centuries ago when he wrote, "We are what we often do. It isn't an action, but rather a habit."

In its most basic form neuroplasticity could be described as a continuous process of making or cutting synapses (neural connections). It's a process in which neurons that are regularly utilized are strengthened, while ones that are less used are cut off. This is where the expression "use it , or you'll lose it' comes into significant meaning.

Chapter 5: Brain Training: Backed Up By Science

Brain training is mostly dependent on the research of brain plasticity, also known as neuroplasticity. The brain's plasticity is its capability to change itself over its lifespan. That means that your brain is always changing. However, whether it's experiencing an improvement or negative one is entirely dependent on your choices, habits and your lifestyle. Thus, the brain training exercises and methods are developed to help you harness this shift and help in increasing your brain's capacity.

In many ways, your brain is the muscle. Both use the same fuel, which is oxygen and glucose. Also they contain neurons. To build muscle, you perform exercises that stimulate the motor neurons within the muscles. Similar to brain training, you can stimulate the brain's neurons to function and process information faster. In the brain, there are around billions of neurons. They are connected via dendrites and axons. They require constant stimulation to remain in top state. You might be thinking that your routine actions like writing, thinking and reading can be enough stimulation for cells to remain in good shape. However, research has proven that a lot the thinking we do on a daily to day basis is not productive since we often create cortisol (a stress hormone that is released by the brain as a response to stress). Cortisol causes brain damage. It destroys the brain cells that reside within the hippocampus (the memory and learning center within the brain). The question is, what activities trigger the development of new neurons? In the past, scientists have suggested activities like crosswords, puzzles and even learning new languages. However, are they really helpful? In a way, yes. Are they the best? Unfortunately, no. Therefore, various techniques for brain training have been devised by top neuroplasticity experts across the globe that anyone can follow to improve their brains.

The methods you'll find in the chapters that follow can be classified in six areas: intelligence Memory, Speed of the brain Navigation, People skills and. Certain of the exercises will help you develop your abilities, while others use an indirect method to improve your basic abilities in sensory perception (for example, spotting objects in a hurry or separating different sounds). This program focuses on the major issues that arise when we age with our brains. The most significant root causes comprise:

A sense of brightness (Slower thinking and reacting in response to events) When we grow older, our brain switch off "brightness". You'll notice that it takes longer to feel alert when you wake up. You might also feel sleepy and fatigued throughout the day, even following having a restful night. Even a restful night isn't enough to revive your vitality as you get older.

The speed of the brain As we the passage of time, our brain decreases in speed, but the external influences do not change.

Light still moves at a normal rate and sounds will remain rapid. In the end, we are unable to remember many things through the entire day. This can make it difficult to recall and react to details we have heard or seen.

Accuracy: With time the neural pathways that are formed inside your brain get fuzzy, blurrier and more scratchy. This makes it harder for the brain keep the details of things and sounds that surround you. The information your brain stores is distorted and unclear.

Recognition: To be able to comprehend something, we must to gather data, piece them up and interpret it. If you don't understand the facial expression of someone else or do not recognize an old acquaintance It's a sign your brain isn't able identify the parts of information. It's true that this is a common issue among older people.

Clarity: Studies have demonstrated that young brains are able to block out background noise and distractions. As we get older and get older, the clarity of the brain decreases. We are unable to concentrate on one thing without becoming distracted halfway through.

Recording: You could be surprised to learn that your brain doesn't always process all data and process it. The neurons inside your brain release neuromodulators, a specific chemical that determine what information is crucial and worthwhile to process. As young as we are neurons release the neuromodulator chemical abundantly, but as we get older, the production rate decreases significantly. In the end, the brain becomes less adept in recording new data and processing the information. In simpler terms the brain becomes slower in recalling, learning and responding.

When the root causes of these issues begin to manifest but we aren't able to recognize them since our brain is adept at filling in the information gaps that aren't being filled with ability to draw inspiration, experience, and context. We draw upon our previous experiences to fill in the gaps and comprehend the information in a way that is not complete. This will help us react quickly in stressful situations however, as time passes and the gaps grow too large to fill in with context, we don't grasp details and act effectively. Therefore, training for the brain is an absolute must for anyone. Studies conducted on the subject of neuroplasticity have proven that brain training can stop these symptoms from showing up and maintain the shape of the brain for longer.

Chapter 6: Practical Routines For

Increased Brain Power

The ability to have a good memory is really dependent on the strength and health of your brain. It doesn't matter whether you're a student an expert, or a older person. There are practical and appropriate ways to follow to improve your brain's capacity. This chapter will show you how. you will be explained how to increase the power of your brain.

A well-known axiom says that new tricks cannot be taught by dogs that are old. However, researchers have proven otherwise. Human brains are remarkably high in terms of adaptability as well as susceptibility to changes. Even when an individual has reached a certain age, they can still be a sponge for learning. This is explained in the term neuroplasticity. If you use the right method to stimulate your brain it will develop new neural pathways. These changes alter the connections within the neuronal network.

The brain adapts and reacts to changes in its environment.

In terms of the capacity to learn and memory the brain displays an exclusive capability, the ability to change its shape and adjust to change. This inherent ability can be utilized if you are looking to improve the capacity to absorb new information, improve your cognitive level, as well as your memory.

The Brain Power Rule #1 Don't miss a workout or sleep.

Like the rest of your body your brain requires certain nutrients in order to perform its job efficiently and at its highest level. This is discussed in detail in the first section of this guide. However, two important aspects of nutrition that must be taken into consideration in this chapter: sleep and exercise.

Are you aware that when you exercise your body, you're also working your brain? Yes. There is studies that demonstrate that there is a direct connection between enhanced cognitive abilities and memory as well as an increased level of exercise.

This is due to the fact that exercise may boost the amount of oxygenation in our brains. Physical activities also reduce the chance of suffering loss of memory or other brain diseases. Additionally, it can help in protection against cardiovascular diseases and diabetes. The most important benefit is that exercise may produce brain chemicals that aid in the defense of neurons.

Additionally, you must take a good amount of rest to be able to function effectively. This will help your brain in working to maximum capacity. If you aren't getting enough sleep, it is likely that you'll be unable to perform of critical thinking capabilities in problem-solving, and your ability to think creatively. Whatever your schedule are, and regardless of the amount of work you have to complete, there's no good reason to avoid sleeping. Sleep deprivation is known as the primary cause for disasters to occur. It is not only important to allow your brain opportunity to relax. It is also crucial to help consolidate memory. Sleep, especially at its most deep levels (which generally occurs in the event of a sufficient amount of sleep) are crucial to the development of memory.

The Brain Power Exercise #2 Don't forget to enjoy yourself and spend some time with your friends

Do you recall the old saying "All work and no play can make you a dull person"? This is real. Being in a serious state every day could "bore" you and your brain. It is not stimulating for creative or critical thought. Spend the time to have some amusement. Take a little bit of time playing the games you enjoy - whether it's on the internet or in the physical world. It is possible to play chess or Candy Crush, but never play for too long playing too much - it could be detrimental to your health as well as your brain. Plan an "me" time: watch movies every once in some time or visit the bar with your buddies. This will provide you with lots of advantages for your brain.

Being social and maintaining a healthy connection with them is vital in order to keep the best health for your body and mind. Remember that humans are social creatures, so your life shouldn't be lived in solitude. The brain is known to be stimulated by connections which are healthy ones. Social interactions with others is the best method of exercising the brain.

Research suggests that forming and maintaining connections that are meaningful improves the brain's health. This creates a robust system of support that can not only improve your mental wellbeing and wellbeing, but also improves your mental well-being. A recent study conducted in a well-known school, it was found that those who have the highest levels of social interaction are less vulnerable to neurodegeneration and decline in memory.

Socialization is often seen as an undervalued task. It offers a number of benefits that improve your memory. If you're in the mood to spare, try to join a group or join a social-civic club. Make sure to visit your friends frequently. If you don't get to meet them, try talking to them on the phone. If you don't have any humans to interact with, at the very least get an animal.

Brain Power Routine #3: Laugh Out Loud

If you haven't realized that, laughter can be extremely beneficial to you as well as your brain. It's not just the most effective medicine for your body but also will also bring benefits to your brain. Other emotional reactions such as anger and crying can affect specific brain regions. However, laughter can be capable of stimulating multiple regions in our brain.

Furthermore, practicing jokes or responding with jokes can serve as a way to stimulate brain areas that are involved in learning and creativity. Where do we begin? Here are the fundamentals of laughing loudly to increase one's emotional intelligence:

Try having fun with yourself. Have fun laughing at the jokes you make yourself. Try sharing your most embarrassing experiences. In this way, you'll be capable of taking yourself less seriously and consider your mistakes as an issue. When you laugh at yourself in some way, you release some of the burden.

Have fun and smile. Join in with the people as they smile. People who are unhappy suppress their natural instincts, which is something it is something you shouldn't do. Learn to accept laughter.

Playing with friends and having fun. The most playful people can have fun and laugh out loud. They laugh at themselves as well as the absurdities of everyday life. They often find a reason to be funny. They are able to laugh with a healthy perception of humor. They don't block out humorous thoughts. Instead, they are able to laugh , and think it to be a contagious phenomenon.

Keep in mind to be light every now and again. It's helpful to keep toys inside your vehicle or in your desk. Perhaps you'd like to display a wall-mounted poster that is humorous to your walls. It's possible to accumulate some comics that are funny as well. You could even put a picture of your family on display at work to remind you that there's always positive reason to be smiling.

Imitate the behavior of children. Be aware of how they go through each day. They are the most healthy heart because they can smile. Take inspiration from their lives which show us the importance of living the world in a positive way and having fun.

Fourth Brain Power Routine Examine your levels of stress

Did you realize that stress could be the most destructive enemy of your brain? As time passes stress (the chronic forms) can damage your brain by destroying one cell at a. It could affect the brain's regions that are associated with memory retrieval and the development and development of brand new memories.

Try the practice of meditation. It is believed to be the most effective strategy to boost the brain's performance by reducing tension. Research has proven that it helps to improve many conditions which affect our well-being. The conditions which can be treated with meditation are: depression, anxiety and chronic pain, diabetes along with hypertension. In addition it can improve your cognitive capabilities by increasing levels of learning, creativity thinking, focus, and concentration.

Meditation is described as magical in that it affects the brain in a variety of ways. According to the images of people who regularly meditate there is more monitoring and recorded on the left side of prefrontal cortex. This brain region is linked to the creation of feelings of calmness and happiness. Brain scans have shown that our cerebral cortex has the capacity to expand its size through regular meditation. The thicker cortex aids in the creation of more neural connections , which are linked to a better ability to remember and improve cognitive abilities.

Additionally, if you want to stay sharp You should stay clear of depression and anxiety. These disorders have detrimental impact on memory. In addition to depression and anxiety stress and worry also impact the brain's activity. If you have one of these issues, most likely, you'll have difficulties recalling important information or making critical decisions and maintaining focus. Therefore, you must maintain your stress levels in control if you wish to enjoy a higher level of mental performance.

Brain Power Routine #5: Engage your brain in an exercise

As you grow older the brain has already created millions and millions of neural pathways. This allows you to sort through the information you are receiving quite quickly. It also lets you solve issues that you know very quickly. Additionally, with no effort from your brain it is possible to perform tasks that are easy to do. Yet, despite all the advancements you've experienced since the beginning it is important to continue stimulating your brain by giving it an exercise every once in the time. This will help it expand and develop. At times it is best to play around with the system.

It is crucial to change the way you conduct your routine. For instance instead of following the same route from office or to the supermarket Why not take an alternative route when you get home? Also, consider exploring different areas on weekends. Every day you should read a book that has a theme of its own. They will all help to stimulate the neurons that are in your brain in a way or another.

The brain's power is available in an "use it or lose it" basis. If you decide to exercise it more, you'll feel that it's easier to process information that is new. Some of the things that can assist you in working out your brain are such as knitting, needlework making pottery or playing tables tennis, juggling as well as playing any instrument. In general, the ability to think, creativity and hand-eye coordination can be improved by these activities.

If you're in search of something new and exciting exercise to stimulate your brain, anything that meets the following qualities is an option

Be sure the exercise is something new to you. Anything that is intellectually challenging is a good training for your brain. If you're already so familiar with it, it will not benefit your brain even by a little. So, you must take the challenge of trying some new things - out of your comfortable zone.

You should make sure you are able to tackle the task. Explore something that can broaden your perspective by acquiring new information. Consider trying a different sport or try a new instrument. If you're not able to find time to play these games, you can try Sudoku or crosswords.

You should ensure that you discover something that you enjoy to engage in. It shouldn't be stress-inducing. Anything that causes stress is unproductive and can make you feel dull. Therefore, you must take pleasure as a primary aspect. In this way, you'll gain more satisfaction from doing what you decide to accomplish.

6. Brain Power Routine: Increase your capacity to recall information and retain

The process of remembering can be difficult for some. If you don't wish to lose the ability to recall information quickly it is advisable try these strategies:

Be attentive to the details. Information that is new won't stick in your mind If you don't be attentive to it. So, if you wish to be able to recall something and retain it later, it's crucial to be focused on the subject. Concentrate on the subject you wish to know for at most 8 seconds. If you don't, you won't be in a position to grasp the concept.

It is easier to do this when you engage your senses. If you're a student trying to pass an exam, you can try chewing gum. When you are taking the test take the same type of gum. This will help you remember what you've learned. This is among the most effective applications of this basic principle. It is possible to include more senses, such as smell, taste and even sight. These senses can assist you in remembering the things you've learned.

Every bit of information must be correlated to your previous knowledge. Connecting the old and new information helps in reducing the amount of effort needed to absorb the details. For example, remembering names of your new acquaintance is much easier if you be able to connect it with the place where you first met them or the way you got to know them.

Concentrate on the basics if you are unable to comprehend something complicated. Do not try to memorize anything you don't know. It will cause stress. Instead, take your time learning by pieces as it helps you master the subject in a an orderly manner.

Chapter 7: Control Mental Fatigue

Have you ever completed the marathon but not completely prepared? Maybe you've decided to get in shape the next day, but were exhausted by the end of your workout. Maybe you picked something that was difficult or you were unaware of how out of shape you were. Mental fatigue can be a lot similar to the latter.

What Is Mental Fatigue

The effects of mental fatigue can occur for a short or long period of time, however the effects are always identical. The brain cells are like tiny muscles and are prone to fatigue from excessive activity. This is similar to the muscles that become stiff after working out extremely hard.

The feeling of tiredness is caused due to a constant level of focus and effort to a specific task along with extreme stress levels. Any process that puts you in overload can cause this problem.

A lot of workers feel fatigued later during the daytime. The tasks they are assigned seem more difficult and complex as well as their focus levels are lower and this leads to more errors being committed. Even nights dedicated to studying or work will make you tired and will eventually result in a negative outcome when you enter the classroom to take the test or presentation that you have did your homework for. You'll be unable to remember anything.

There's no solution for this condition and although there are many herbal remedies that are available for energy boost, they're not permanent and may cause more damage in the long run. There are a variety of ways you can aid yourself even if you're suffering from fatigue in your mind.

The most effective way to reduce cognitive fatigue is through exercising. Exercise can increase the amount of oxygen that flows through your bloodstreams. This improves your mental performance. Another way to combat mental fatigue is to alter your diet. It's not so much your weight that's the issue It's the quantity of nutrition you're receiving. The brain thrives on food and when your body is healthy then your brain is also healthy.

It's not unusual to see people eat a sweet snack early in the day, then smoke cigarettes, and sip an espresso before heading off to work. In starting their mornings in this manner, people are setting themselves up to indulge in a sugary meal and then smoking cigarettes throughout the day. Although sugar can give them some energy but it's only temporary and can cause problems later in the day. The cycle is that you get energetic, then abruptly dropping off, only to consume and drink sugar or caffeine to feel energized once more. This vicious cycle wears down your cognitive abilities because you're not in a state of equilibrium.

The best way to combat physical fatigue is to choose an appropriate diet that is balanced and full of nutrients, not sugar or caffeine. A diet with plenty of vegetables and fruits in it is a great start.

How to Battle Mental Fatigue - Tips and Strategies for Battling Mental Fatigue and Pushing Forward

Balance

The first thing to be aware of about mentally fatigue is that it is an fact that nutrition plays a significant role in it. You must eat a nutritious breakfast or lunch and dinner to fight fatigue in your mind. However, that doesn't mean you do not stop.

It is also important to have a restful night's sleep however that doesn't necessarily be eight hours for you. Some people are content with just six hours. One way to determine how many hours you'll need to rest in the night is to fall asleep in the evening when you are exhausted on weekends and then get up when you feel at ease at the beginning of the day. You can count the amount of time you've slept. This is how much sleep you'll require for sleep.

If you've not had any physicals in a while You might want to talk to your doctor regarding how much vitamin you have.

Certain deficiencies can lead to fatigue and it's hard to tell if that we're lacking in vitamins if we weren't tested for blood.

Brain Drain Remedy

There's a famous Zen story of two monks. Each day they walk whole day to the temple. On their way to the temple, they're unable to talk or communicate with other people particularly women. On one occasion, the monk comes across a woman who is standing in a river, struggling to traverse the river. He takes her by the hand and then carries she across the water while the other monk stares in shock.

The second monk doesn't say anything to the monk who is the first and they continue to walk. Three hours after the second monk is unable to contain his anger longer, and shouts to one monk "How could you pick up that woman?" The second monk replies: "I held that woman for five minutes - you've been carrying her for three hours."

The lesson is that you're in the choice of the burdens you carry around with you , if there are any. In the event that you're carrying it around your attention isn't paid your friends, family or even you. You're too caught up in what's happened in the past, instead of looking at the present.

Getting Rid of Negativity

The reality of our lives is that emotions can be transmitted. There are neurons in our brains that reflect the emotions of others. People with the classification of empathic actually have more neurons than other. We're taught to perceive the emotions of other people through our brains which is why it's acceptable to be around negative people? Researchers say no.

You should restrict your interactions with negative people If you are unable to manage to stay away from them, let them know how they're making your feel.

Another aspect of negativity is being in a position to say"no" to people. There are times when we have a million things to accomplish in a single day, and that's because we were unable to say no to the day before. Make a decision about what is the most important to you and let go of other things to do.

Qigong Breath

Qigong breath is an ancient yoga practice that relies on meditation and visualization. To do the practice sit with your feet aligned with your hips, and bring your hands at your sides. As you breathe, lift your arms towards the sides, palms facing upwards until they're overhead. Now imagine that energy is that is above you and you are accumulating it with your hands and feel it in your arms. After exhaling, imagine you're sending that energy into the earth. Visualize it in the form of a golden glow that cleanses and relaxes your body as it passes through your body. Repeat this three times.

Love Blast

Imagine your face with someone who you cherish or admire even if you don't have someone think of your pet. Anything you truly love. When you do this, you're releasing endorphins in your body that provide you with an energy boost.

Chapter 8: Mindfulness

As we near the conclusion in this adventure, I would like to believe you've gained a lot of knowledge regarding yourself, the way you feel feelings and the way you think. to think on a regular basis. I hope that you are acquainted with the places as well as the experiences you have that cause thinking too much. The technique we discussed over in the past is a great technique to stop the cycle of thinking too much, and establishing healthy, new habits that you can practice on a regular basis is a fantastic method to change those old routines that are no longer useful.

There's plenty to get out of fresh air in a park , or even reading a book instead of overloading your mind with irrelevant and depressing social media or news feeds. You've been able to deal with the negative influences that have impacted your life from friends to magazines and are beginning becoming a brand new person, ready to pursue your desires. I hope that you've also gained some knowledge about your chosen job or career choice and, even though it's likely to be the most difficult area to alter I hope you've either confirmed your happiness and contentment in your current position or taken the first steps toward making a decision that's specific to your abilities and what you love about your job.

The final thing I'd like introduce during this article is about mindfulness. There are three types of mindfulness that I'd like to explore, but they're all related and form a part of one another. In general, I would like to discuss all three as they're often interchangeable and even if you don't recognize any of them, you've heard of a different. They're mindfulness meditation, meditation and positive thinking.

It's true that you might think that positive thinking isn't exactly the same as mindfulness or meditation, however in many ways, I believe positive thinking as an aspect of meditation, and I'll explain it in a little. Let's first understand mindfulness more clear.

Mindfulness

When I mention the term "mindfulness," many people typically think of the term "paying attention." If this is the thought you were thinking of, you're not wrong! Attention to what you're doingin your surroundings as well as how you're feeling is a crucial aspect of being mindful. However, it's more than simply paying attention and for many it's more challenging than it seems.

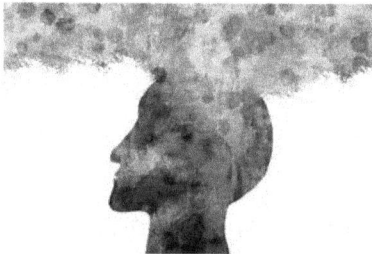

Mindfulness is the practice of being present, not only for a few minutes however, all day, every day, for the duration throughout your entire life. It is important to keep your awareness all the time although we all recognize that we aren't machines or computers and there will be occasions that we become distracted or our minds get flooded with emotions and thoughts which take us off as we react to events in our lives. The parallels can be drawn from a religious perspective. In the Christian philosophy, followers acknowledge that they are humans and may make mistakes, while trying their best to live a sin-free holy, righteous and a faithful life. We all know that we'll make mistakes isn't a reason to not try. This is why the lasting effects on our lives physically, spiritually and even physically are worth the effort. So, let's examine the benefits that mindfulness can offer us and then discover how to integrate mindfulness into your daily life.

Imagine the way you feel when you've successfully eliminated a negative or harmful thought, in exchange for a fresh positive thought. It makes you feel good, right? Also, it gives you the feeling of being clear, as if a huge mess was just cleaned off the floor in your head. It's the same when we begin to be mindful. With mindfulness, is there the added benefit.

The practice of mindfulness regularly leads to a sense of potential or hope and of looking ahead with fresh eyes. It is a time to move ahead with an open head and taking note of every moment that passes your way. When I speak about a sense of possibility and looking ahead to the future, I'm not talking about anticipating the next weekend, day, or even a month. It's about taking steps forward, one step at a time day by day experiencing and observing everything surrounding you and feeling each second as it passes. You will feel a sense of satisfaction and happiness that comes as you get rid of thoughts that are not useful to you in the present. Your mind is thanking you.

Your soul and heart are grateful to you. There's so much to feel and be thankful for right now. Mindfulness is all about shifting into focus this intimate and small-scale approach to thinking. And in this way, your entire world is revealed to you.

How can you begin practicing mindfulness? It's true that the most difficult task in this case will be improving your ability to staying focused. However, there's a bright side. If you've managed to use the interruption technique to change your negative thoughts and feelings by positive thoughts and emotions, you've been able to develop this ability. Focus is the effort to sharpen your thinking skills and narrowing the task down to one task, without letting your thoughts wander off to thoughts that aren't aiding you in completing the task. Like I've said earlier, you don't want to get caught in the trap of striving so much that this exercise becomes a burden and cause of anxiety for you. Anyone who is brand new and is just beginning to learn about mindfulness will progress and grow in a different way since we are all unique humans. This is perfectly normal. Just like the other topics that's in the book, the most important thing is to start small at one time.

A great way to exercise mindfulness is to take a walk and be in the natural world.

Take a walk in the park that is peaceful and sit on a bench or at a picnic table. Relax for a while and relax your mind. Take some time to achieve this. As you focus your thoughts, pay attention to the sounds around you, dogs barking or the breeze moving in the branches. Feel the breeze blowing on your face, or the sunlight's heat pounding down on your body. Feel your body floating in space. Make sure that you're sitting in a comfortable posture. Close your eyes when you begin. As you begin to focus and appreciate on what's happening around you then slowly let your eyes open. Take in the things you see, without having thoughts about them. It's possible that this won't be a natural thing, but it will become easier through practice. Be aware of the beauty of your surroundings no matter what it is that you notice. If you don't have a beautiful park nearby You can perform the same thing in your backyard or even in your neighborhood. Pay attention to the birds, or children playing on the street. Make an effort to concentrate on experiences without thinking about them, or letting your mind wander. If you can be mindful for only a few minutes every day, you'll begin to notice it becoming more effortless the more you do it.

Meditation

Discussions on mindfulness flow naturally into a discussion about meditation, since they are connected. According to me, they're both a part of one another and are a way of describing different practices.

Meditation, for many means being mindful throughout the day every day. For others, it's the time that is set aside each week or day that is utilized for regular meditation practices that are based on an individual philosophical or thought-based school. For example, Zen Buddhism. I will also mention different types of meditation, but I will focus on Zen specifically since it is the type of meditation with which I am the most comfortable.

The same techniques you've used in nature are a great way to incorporate them into a exercise in meditation. Since the majority of people think of meditation as the idea being in a peaceful space while keeping your eyes shut, lets take a look at ways you can begin to practice meditation in your home with the steps below.

Based on your ability Find a comfortable spot in which you can sit comfortably with your back fairly straight. The arms must be at your sides and your neck shouldn't be stretched. A quick Google search will show the formal seating structure If you're interested but for now we'll take an informal approach to the physical posture and concentrate on what's happening within your head.

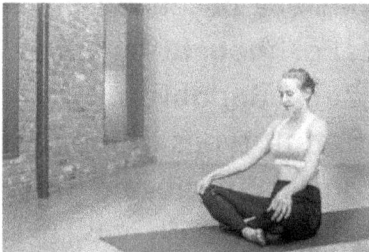

When we talked about mindfulness, we spoke about taking in the world around us and paying attention to what is happening to you at the present moment. Meditation is similar to that, with the exception that in the practice that is Zen mindfulness, the objective is not to limit your thoughts, but to avoid focusing on specific thoughts that enter and out of your mind. The primary goal is to concentrate on the present moment, however the premise of Zen is to not enclose the mind, but instead allow the mind to be free and let it flow as it returns to the present.

For example, have noticed yourself or a loved one was able to catch you staring at the ceiling looking at the ceiling at the screen as your mind wanders off and begins to engage in an argument with yourself about an incident from recently or something you may have committed in the past? The process of thinking is taking you off the present and now you're immersed in the replay of events that were already past and can't be changed. Yet, you continue to focus on those instances as if they were mistakes, and worry about what others think of you, but the truth is that they aren't aware of those small incidents. Are you familiar with this?

It's not uncommon to do it. The main goal of meditation is to stay clear of those thoughts that do to drag us out of our present in the past or future, which are either unchangeable or are not changeable or can't be predicted. The brain loves to learn things and make patterns in attempt to predict and comprehend our lives. However, we can get caught into this obsession until we don't see life as it is right now.

Zen is all about acknowledging the wandering nature of the mind but also accepting the core principle of impermanence--everything changes, even the thoughts in your mind. Concentrating on one idea, feeling or thought is pointless and insignificant to an ever-changing world. It will keep you in a stalemate.

This might not make sense right now, but when you're trying to get started at the beginning look back to the sentence we discussed at the very beginning of this chapter.

Simply "pay attention." Look around, feel your body in space, pay attention, and appreciate. It's all you have to be focusing on to start. Similar to all positive practices, you'll quickly develop a new dependence on the happiness that mindfulness brings. Following this, mindfulness will come naturally.

Like I mentioned earlier meditation can come in various forms and it is important to not believe that there is only one method to practice meditation. Many people practice mindfulness and mediation through music and movement, a process known as dance meditation. Others, like Zen Buddhist monks, practice "walking meditation." Movement is often a way to calm and regulate the mind when we create movements that are like our free-flowing thoughts. Whatever style or preference you have keep in mind the reason you're doing it in the first place. And there are no excuses for "doing it wrong."

Positive Thinking

Positive thinking has a lot to do with the technique of thinking where we interrupted negative thoughts and replacing them with positive ones. However, with positive thinking the goal is to build positive thoughts first instead of waiting for them to be used and then using them to counteract negative thoughts. Another method of practice can look different from one individual to individual. It should also not be an overly complex and prevent anyone from doing it.

Simply simply, positive thinking is when that you get up each day and contemplating each day as a brand exciting, and unpredictable day instead of worrying about what you believe is likely to occur. There is no way to predict the future even if your daily routine appears to be fixed in stone, if you start to get into the habit of worrying about every day something related the work environment (which is something I'm sure you've already tackled!) and then you shut yourself off from experiencing exciting items or events that make you smile. It's possible to understand the concept I'm talking about by using an illustration.

Consider Mr. Scrooge from the classic Christmas story, "A Christmas Carol." It's Christmas Eve and children are laughing while playing outside in snow. and people buying gifts for Christmas and chatting with strangers. However, there's Scrooge. Scrooge trudging through the snow towards the office. He's already thinking the Christmas season is horrible season and there's no joy in it. There is only loss of cash. Since he's determined that he won't be having a good time at Christmas, he's in no position to be open to the joy being experienced everywhere.

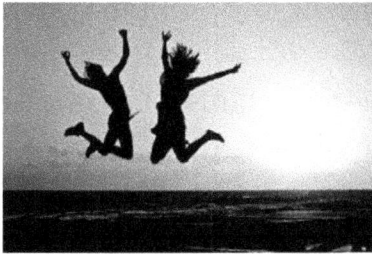

In the same way, when we wake up and are worried about what's going to happen the following day, we are blind to events that could bring joy, surprise, and joy.

Have you ever thought about how people get subtle signals to not engage or communicate with you when you're unhappy or upset? Consider all the enjoyable conversation you've had with friends at work when you're with a positive attitude positive and open to whatever your day might be throwing at you. This thought can serve as an inspiration to strive to cultivate positive thoughts every single day, starting in the beginning of each day.

Cultural Backing for the Effects of Positive Thinking
You might or may not be aware that is known as"the "law of attraction" as it was popularized in films such as The Secret. People think that thinking positively helps to bring positive things and results on your life if you consistently practice it. It's likely that you've heard the expression, "if you put your mind to it, you can accomplish anything." That's what positively thinking, and law of attraction are all about.

It can be helpful to write about your experiences as you master this ability. Make a list of goals to achieve in your life. Perhaps it's something that you've been thinking about for years and years or perhaps it's something you've been thinking about for a while. Make a note of your goal in your journal. Write some notes about the way to achieve it. be like for you. Maybe you envision yourself and your family and people at a huge celebration for the news of a promotion, or perhaps you've arranged for your family to go on a trip in the Bahamas. Perhaps you're picturing you've lost 30 pounds in that brand new bathing suit that you've had an eye for a long time. Whatever the reason this is the goal to document your experience in the most detail you can. Make the experience real in your head Then write down what you observe.

The next step is note down the steps that will be on the path to your desired goal. Positive thinking can be a powerful tool, but in order to make your dream a reality, you'll be required to put in the effort.

What are you required to accomplish between now and next year to aid you in achieving your goal? What strategy do you have that you can follow to lose weight in a safe and sustainable manner that you will be able to sustain?

If you've ever watched any of the film awards shows, you might recognize the speeches that winners of the show give where they admit to dreaming and contemplating their goals for years before they could actually achieve the goals they set for themselves.

If you allow yourself to become depressed and believe that you'll never achieve something, then it is likely that you aren't going to succeed. Positive thinking can naturally lead you toward your objectives since you are urging your self, both subconsciously and consciously to be ready for the opportunities you could be unable to see with a negative outlook. Like Scrooge and his insanity to joy, it's also possible to be encased with negativity so tightly that you are unable to see an opportunity in the front of you.

Be mindful and positive by taking small steps every day. Soon it will be easy and natural to keep going. The satisfaction and happiness which comes from practicing this is something that your mind as well as your body and soul will soon begin to desire. Similar to when you workout and your body recompenses you for all the positive emotions from endorphins as well as an overall feeling of achievement your body and mind will reward you with positive emotions in the near future. It becomes difficult to resist the urge to be positive.

Don't rely on me to prove it. If you're determined to maintain and cultivate the positive changes you've made within your daily life, certain that you'll hear about it from your closest friends as they observe the transformations taking place. They may even be inspired to study more about mindfulness as well as meditation and positive thinking to make these methods essential to their lives, too.

In the final chapter of our series we'll be talking about the importance of rest in your daily life. As a last thought and an instrument to learn from this journey, I hope that you will do all possible to facilitate your sleep simpler, including taking a rest each night for a reasonable period of. A good night's sleep could mean the most important factor in determining success or failure, because it has significant impact on the way that the brain performs in the long and short term. Let's find out some more about the importance sleep plays in and how it is related to the daily routines that we live our life.

Chapter 9: Brain Fitness Training

The importance of educating the mind to improve its fitness level is becoming increasingly popular. The brain training program is an established set of methods created to increase your brain power. The courses test your memory, reasoning and ability to visualize. It can be extremely beneficial for people who struggle with disorders or mental issues.

A successful brain fitness program starts by assessing your cognitive abilities. This is important to determine any weaknesses that you require to improve by with the methods included in the program. Cognitive abilities that need assessment include auditory and visual processing, speed of processing in reasoning and logic as well as memory and attention span.

Your test results will be evaluated with the director of your course, who will suggest a suitable program to correct your deficiencies based on the results of the assessment. If you are in agreement, the next step, which is the actual training is followed.

There are websites offering brain-training courses within the comforts of your home if you don't want to take advantage of formal fitness programs. They provide brain-training exercises along with games and activities that can be both enjoyable and demanding.

The goal of these exercise routines is to aid you process your information quickly and efficiently. They also improve your ability to multitask if required. They improve your ability to focus and concentrate on crucial tasks. They boost your speed of remember things and events.

You can personal develop your brain through:

Memory challenge - Test yourself to memorize the lyrics of the latest song. Use your left hand to perform something , even if you're right-handed or dressed in the dark. When you perform your daily chores in a different way or by purchasing different ones done, your level of acetylcholine of your brain is increased. This chemical can create brain cells and enhance your memory.

Attention problem As you get older, your attention span diminishes, and multi-tasking becomes more challenging. It is possible to increase your ability to focus by trying to make your brain work by combining two different activities simultaneously. For instance, you can solve math problems while running or reading an audio book as you drive to home. Another method that works is to change the routine you are used to, like changing your work table. The idea is to make your brain to pay attention and get used to this new pattern.

Language test - Read more than your normal reading material and if you discover words that are completely new to you, write them down, and then search for the definition within the Dictionary. While you work on this practice of understanding the context behind the words you've learned you're building your skills in the language and increasing your vocabulary.

It also increases your fluency and grammatical understanding.

Physical and Spatial Challenge - Test your skills to walk around in the room, then choose five items and remember their places. Continue with your normal task, but after an hour, remember what the items are and where they're located. This activity forces your brain to trigger your memory and concentrate on what is happening in your surroundings. You could also take note of five things while waiting for your ride , and remember them later. Keep doing this until you're comfortable with the items you find at your specific location.

Executive Brain Functions Challenge - These are tasks which require you to create an action plan to reach your goal and take the right decisions to reach it quickly. For instance, you can play games on video. It is a strategy that must be well-planned to prevail against a foe whether human or virtual. It is based on the power of reasoning, logic, and decision-making abilities.

Mind Mapping Challenge - It makes use of brainstorming to tackle problems. It involves writing the primary idea on an article of paper and surrounding it with a circle and then writing down a variety of options to solve the issue. Connect them with lines to the primary issue. Write down every possibilities. This is the creative mind at work. You can then analyze your strategies before choosing the strategy to use in solving the problem.

Chapter 10: Physically

One of the most difficult things to attain that people acknowledge is attempting to lose weight. Being at an appropriate weight, and not just look good, but also feeling healthy often escapes the majority of people. This is the reason that the greatest amount of gym commitments as well as contracts signed during the initial two weeks of the season (January-February). We are aware that staying physically fit should be our top priority, yet we do not have the ability to achieve this ideal.

Because of our American typical diet that is comprised of a large amount of carbohydrates and sugars as well as fats which fuels the scourge of the perpetual condition of health deterioration. With all of these issues that hinder our ability to stay fit and healthy by eating a balanced diet and regularly physical activity, how can get our health back to its peak levels? If you've answered "by focusing on your brain" and you're right, then you've got the correct solution.

Move!

One of the most significant consequences of our ever-growing technological and scientific knowledge is the huge improvement in our lives as humans as compared to the past century. We drive cars instead of horses, we're using smartphones instead of writing letters (even although it's useful) We have chairs all over the place, which means we're not standing all the all of the time.

The unsettling truth of our rapid advancement in technology is that every activity we engage in is a reflection of our strengths and its own challenges. The battles with the world we've constructed through our minds is that our lifestyle of sedentary is not the primary causes for your parasympathetic nerve response to becoming hyperactive, and to respond in a dangerous and unpredictable manner. Because the process is controlled by your brain, that means these areas of the brain are losing certain functions because of a lack of active lifestyle.

Listen, when I say "non-active", I am not talking about attending the gym at least four times per week for 2 hours at a time. It is simply living a life that involves basic act of standing and walking around for 10 minutes per hour of sitting. To reduce or even reverse the negative effects the lifestyle of sedentary has to your brain you must be active and up. Do something, anything! This is not just good to your mind, it is is vital to ensure the continuous maximum performance of it too.

Another thing that your brain enjoys is exercising vigorously enough to produce sweat. According to Jim Kwik, when your body moves, your brain is in a groove. Training that causes sweat can also help your brain to grow younger. It will release the right amount of dopamine which is the motivating chemical and releases BDNF which aids in learning things more quickly. When you make your body abrasive to improve your brain's strength.

It is not necessary to do a two-hour workout to sweat. It's as easy as doing the High-Intensity Interval Training (HIIT for short). What exactly is it? It's about choosing three to four exercises and completing each one without stopping. If you finish each of the four exercises, that amounts to one round. An ideal HIIT set will take three to four rounds.

Example: 10 pull-ups 15 push-ups 20 squats 25 sit-ups, three rounds. The rounds are non-stop between rounds and exercises.

The primary benefit of this kind of exercise is that it allows you to get the most amount of output for only a small amount of input. The primary input you provide is the intensity. A complete HIIT session should not run more than 25 minutes, however, you will still reap the advantages of a 60-minute aerobic exercise. In order to reap the benefits of a workout lasting 60 minutes in only 25 minutes, three times per week is a less expensive decision rather than spending all day at the gym for a standard exercise.

Eat Right

With burgers, wings and fried food everywhere we go, it's quite impossible to be healthy. However, even if we attempt to eat properly, we aren't able to make the right choices as we're plagued by cognitive fog as well as low levels of energy and a crash following each meal. This isn't routine. When you consume food, it's meant to help you wake up to bring clarity and provide you with energy. It is supposed to provide fuel for our bodies and not be being a burden that holds us back from doing our most optimal.

So, what kinds of food do we consume? Which are the most beneficial to my brain? Before we get into the foods that can help you start your path to better health, it is important to know that trying to eat a diet that will benefit your waistline is not worth your time. Foods that claim to reduce your stomach's size may be detrimental to the other parts in your physique. If you put your brain into the focus everyone else is rewarded.

In the process of beginning our journey towards a healthier and more powerful brain, it is important to realize something that is contrary to all the information you've been given fat is healthy for your health, while sugar can be the primary source of bad health. The thing to consider is that the body may not require the amount of sugar you might think, and that's even if it comes from natural sources.

If you eat protein, your body goes through the process of gluconeogenesis which means that your body creates sugar (energy) to fuel your muscle. In the end, you don't need to consume a lot of sugar, if at all, to be able to function on energy. This is a lie that popular media has propagated to people.

Another lie they've propagated is the demonization of fat. Fat isn't evil. Actually, the majority parts of your grey matter are comprised of fat. It is essential to consume the right saturated fats to have a strong and strong brain. If you consume higher quantities of fat, and cut down on carbohydrates, your liver releases ketones. They are the most pure source of energy that your brain makes use of. Ketone-powered brains are ones that is extremely clear, with unlimited quantities of energy, as well as the complete elimination of brain fog.

Foods that are rich in saturated fats and low in sugars/carbs, as well as free from trans fat (the fat that's bad for your body and mind) are the ones your brain will be thankful for. Avocados, grass-fed protein and grass-fed ghee and butter can make your brain dance. Avoid cakes, breads juices, or other sweet fruits like bananas.

If cleaning the entire area of your pantry is not feasible I would suggest to take baby steps. Start by eating your lunch using the items mentioned above. Begin with what you have and not what you aren't able to.

The benefit when you eat more fats is your body uses fat for energy instead of carbs. Due to this shift in the energy source it is possible to use more fat. Fat is healthy for you!

If you get off your desk and walk around, sweat little and eat right foods to fuel your brain, you'll notice a dramatic improvement in your health, waistline and your body. You'll begin to feel more youthful and experience more confidence as a result of your appearance. When you concentrate upon your mind, it will repay you.

Chapter 11: How To Increase Your Brain Power With Brain Training

Knowing all this, it's simple to see how brain-training can be effective in theory by helping you build more connections in your brain and also to make new ones completely - thus making new connections and enhancing the ones you already are already proficient in.

This is the reason that has led to the creation of many brain-training websites and programs that train how to go about doing maths tests or even memory-related challenges. The more you practice this (in the theory) the better you develop your skills, and the better your memory, attention span or mental math will improve.

This is like a seal of approval! Then, should you proceed and begin using this kind or brain-training?

I argue no. While games such as Lumocity and Nintendo Brain Age might be helpful in testing your memory or your unique perception, the truth is that they're far too limited to be all suitable in real life. If you practice to be more adept at recognizing the number of adorable penguins in a crowd (this is the type of setting that these brain-training games frequently offer) and you get more adept at this. The brain is strengthened by neural connections with penguins. It's a game that you repeat time and time again, and getting better at the game, but it's not going to help your ability to formulate responses to an interview. It's not transferrable to "real world' abilities and, as such it won't prove useful.

What is the best way to learn to be more confident in interviews? Simple: give yourself more interviews! This puts you in the exact conditions you require to develop your skill, and ensure that you're using the correct neural pathways.

But that's not to suggest the entire brain-training process isn't worth the time...

The Very Best Form of Brain Training

The most effective method of brain training it to push your self to do a variety of cognitive tasks, and to constantly expose yourself to different situations and problems.

Also you must constantly explore new ideas, constantly try new things and push your brain to continue expanding. The more you work out your brain's ability to adapt the simpler it will become and the greater amount of dopamine, norepinephrine and brain-derived neurotrophic factor, and so on. you'll produce.

It's the moment you quit learning about new things and stop pushing oneself that your mind begins to become very inactive and begins to lose your abilities.

Brain plasticity is able to work in two ways. Pruning can occur in the event that you are for an extended period of time without using a particular neural pathway. This is the reason why we are prone to lose things over time. Additionally, the brain eventually stops producing neurotransmitters that increase neuroplasticity. Brain-derived neurotrophic factors (BDNF) along with dopamine is both directly linked to neurogenesis and myelination (the formation of brain cells) however, if you don't utilize them, they'll appear less frequently.

A happy and healthy brain are brains that you use in a variety of different ways.

Imagine what an incredible child you were as a newborn. What is the reason? It is partly because everything around you is unique.

The world is full of things that aren't understood by you and your brain is inundated with neurochemicals that help make sense of everything.

As you grow older as you age, connections become more established and you get to know the world around you more. However, you'll be learning different things, and experiencing plenty of new experiences. This includes when you attend college and school, when you return home, as you grow older and begin driving, or when you explore new activities...

However, you then reach the age of adulthood. You have a satisfying relationship then you find an occupation you enjoy and your life begins to find the rhythm. The same job you have every day and night out, for the next 50 years. As you age more limited are the chances to explore new ideas you've had. You remain with the same group of friends and you continue to engage in the same interests... And your mind slows down.

This could cause danger in the future when you are more susceptible to experiencing dementia-related cognitive decline as you age or conditions like dementia or Alzheimer's. In addition you'll become more sluggish and more accustomed to your routines and less able to develop new skills.

And that's one reason why we see that our fluid intelligence (intelligence rather than knowledge) is diminished as we age.

It doesn't need to be this way! It's not if you know the importance of constantly expose yourself to new experiences and keep on learning.

Learn new languages constantly. Discover new games. Meet new people. Explore new destinations.

Just being in a new environment can result in a surge of neurotransmitters related to awareness and attention to go off. Find different ways to get home from work! Take a walk and wander around.

Make use of your body training with your body is exactly the purpose that brains are built for, as we've observed and it's an extremely important method to challenge your self and keep on improving your knowledge.

Find activities that give your brain useful'skills in addition. If you're trying to get more out of your brain Why not try learning other languages to can process more information? Do you want to improve your math skills? Or learn programming?

The irony is that these kinds of things will prove to be more beneficial when it comes to an even better memory!

The Power of Computer Games

It might be surprising to you how effective computer games can be the process of to boosting your brain's power.

At one point, we believed computer games were not good for kids, that they would destroy their brains, making them violent (or some other thing). But the reality is more different.

Computer games are now studied in research studies to help improve the ability to make decisions under pressure.

Shooting with action guns allows players to make better decisions faster than those who don't engage in computer games. Additionally they can improve your the visual acuity of our eyes - making us more effective at noticing the differences in colors and seeing things in the distance (which obviously is due to watching out for targets). Computer games may also increase the chances of having lucid dreams which is a form of dreaming in which you are aware that you're asleep , and acquire an ability to regulate your movement and the contents of your dream!

However, that's not the only place where the true power of computer games is. Computer games provide an entirely new type of brain-training because every game is distinct. Each game has different controls, and teaches our motor skills in different ways. Each game exposes us to brand new 3D worlds. Sometimes, even the physics alter!

Every time you start the latest game, you're asked to understand the new controls as well as the new rules. It's time to begin finding how to navigate in the new world and must change your thinking. It all depends on plasticity, because new neural networks are created in your motor cortex and the prefrontal cortex.

When you master an entirely new game, you're mastering the new skills. You'll experience the same dopamine releases (moreso actually) once you've got the right answer!

The reality is more compelling than it appears. The games we play on our computers can be addictive due to releases of dopamine. What triggers the release of dopamine during games? It's because we're learning. The brain loves to learn and if you're able to make learning enjoyable, then it's not long before you'll be more proficient in all things!

Chapter 12: How To Perform

Popular Brain Exercises

The calves pump is a well-known exercise to strengthen the brain. It will help increase your focus, concentration as well as your comprehension. It will also let you complete tasks with more energy.

For this exercise in your brain, simply sit in front of the wall and place the hands of your shoulders. Spread your left leg out behind you, and allow your foot reach the floor. Your heel should not touch the floor, and your entire body needs to be tilted at 45 degrees.

Exhale and lean back against the wall. Flex your left knee, then press your left heel to the floor. Breathe deeply and lift your body up. Relax and then raise your left leg. Repeat this process for at minimum three times switching your legs.

A different exercise that is ideal for you are cook's hook-ups. It connects the two brain hemispheres and increase the electrical energy that your body produces.

This is a great exercise when you are in stressful situations. It will also boost your self-confidence and increase your energy level.

For this exercise, be sitting on a chair and rest your left foot on your left knee. Hold your left ankle with your right hand, and then grab your ball on the left foot using your left hand.

Inhale, and then put your tongue in the roof of your mouth. Place it flatly about a quarter centimeter behind the teeth. Relax your tongue when you exhale. After that, shut your eyes and remain in this position for four to eight minutes.

Slowly return your legs to the position you were in before. Your feet should be level across the ground. After that, bring your hands in a gentle manner as if you were wrapping an object. The eyes must remain shut. Your tongue should be lifted when you inhale , and decrease it as you exhale. Keep this position for approximately 4-8 breaths.

There are also the earth button and the brain button. Earth buttons activate your mind and help relieve it of mental fatigue. Additionally, it may help you focus on the things you need to focus.

For this exercise, place your two fingers below your lower lips. The fingertips of the other hand on your navel, and then point your fingers towards the downwards. Take a deep breath as you gaze at the floor, then move your eyes slowly from the floor to the ceiling before returning down towards the ground. Repeat this process for at least three times.

Brain buttons On the other hand are able to stimulate your carotid arteries , which supply fresh oxygenated blood to the brain. This exercise helps to restore the directional signals from various parts within your body and brain. It will also help enhance your reading, writing and speaking skills, as well as your ability to follow instructions.

For this exercise, just place your finger onto your navel. Use your thumb and fingers of the opposite hand, to sense the hollow spots under your collarbone. Be sure to rub them vigorously for 30 seconds to a minute as you move you head to the left or right.

Chapter 13: What Is Neuroplasticity?

What you learn in this book will transform your life

You're going to embark on an exciting journey through the field of neuroplasticity. Within this section, you'll be taught the meaning of "neuroplasticity" means, along with a basic understanding of brain terms to help you comprehend what's happening in the brain when you are learning an entirely new skill or increase your understanding. You'll be taken on brief overview of the fascinating research psychologists have conducted that shows that neuroplasticity is an amazing process that's discovered in various groups in numerous research studies. Learn what you can do to benefit from these findings to enhance your life in general, your capacity to learn, and even aiding in regulating your mood. It will be clear the reasons why your main priority should be addressing your sleeping habits and diet to take full benefit of your amazingly flexible brain.

What is "neuroplasticity"?

In its simplest form definition "neuroplasticity" refers to the brain's capacity to change. The brains we have aren't just chunks of gray matter inertly that reside in our skulls. They are active organs that are constantly developing throughout the early weeks of life until the time of death. Every time you interact your environment or engage in a particular activity, the right pathways are strengthened within your brain. The most important message from this book is If you alter your behavior and think, you will be able to make massive leaps in the development of your capabilities as an individual. Neuroplasticity research has allowed doctors, academics and all those looking to improve their self-development, to take an positive view of the our potential to grow and development at any age. If you're looking to live a more fulfilled and more productive lifestyle and who wouldn't want to? Learning about neuroplasticity and the applications it has can be a good place to begin.

The basics of brain science

In order to fully comprehend neuroplasticity it is essential to know the basics of neuroplasticity and terminology. There aren't a lot! To maximize the value of this book there are a few bits of background information that you should be aware of.

In the beginning, it's beneficial to learn a of the ways the brain works. When you think of the brain, you'll probably think of the outer layer, the one that appears wrinkled and gray. The scientific name used for this part of the brain is known as the cerebrum. It is divided into two halves, referred to as cerebral hemispheres. Underneath the gray surface (also called "gray matter") there is a white area, also known by the name of "white matter." Most researchers agree that it's the cerebrum that defines us as human. It allows us to reflect as well as learning as well as other cognitive processes. The cerebrum is generally healthy (with some wrinkles) in species of animals that are known for their intelligence such as elephants, dolphins and non-human primates like Chimpanzees.

The way your brain is structured
Within the cerebrum, there are four regions, or lobes. These are:

Frontal Lobe: This helps us make plans and make decisions. It helps us think about the future, defergrate and act in a manner that is responsible. They don't stop developing until we reach our 20s and this helps in the reason why adolescents and children generally have a difficult time learning to see the future, and take sound long-term decisions.
Parietal Lobe: This helps us to pay attention to our surroundings . It is also accountable for our spatial perception. The parietal lobe assists you to find a new spot or catch a ball and feel what something is like.

Temporal Lobe helps us to perceive the meaning of language, to make sense the sounds we make and also to draw upon the auditory memory of our past.

Occipital Lobe: This helps us process and use visual information. To truly appreciate what's happening all around you and to fully appreciate the world around you, you not only require a pair of active eyes, but you also need in a position to comprehend the meaning of all this sensory information. The occipital lobe helps you to do this.

The beautiful brain cells of the brain

There are a variety of cells that compose the human brain. However, the most important type to be considered when discussing neuroplasticity is neurons. They are the ones responsible for transmitting messages throughout the brain through electrical and chemical signals. There are approximately 85 billion neurons within the human brain. Each neuron is capable of connecting around 10,000 times to other neurons. This is an enormous number of connections that could be made! Neurons begin developing in one month in human existence. An embryo develops 250,000 neurons per minute. The rapid growth of neurons is called neurogenesis. In the past, it was thought that neurogenesis ended around in childhood, however, it turns out that brains are able to create new neurons throughout the course of our lives.

Between our neurons, we have synapses. They are tiny gaps that permit the two neurons exchange through these electrical or chemical signals. When we are born, we have around 2500 synapses. This grows to 15,000 by 3 years old.

A shift in perspective - the way that scientists have changed their views on neuroplasticity

As mentioned previously the idea of neuroplasticity is thrilling because for a long time, it was believed humans' brains would never change after a person was at a certain point in their physical development. What led scientists to think it was a fixed brain, an piece of machinery which was not capable of growth or expansion?

In the beginning, those suffering from brain injuries rarely recuperate from the injuries. For instance, neurologist Paul Broca observed that most sufferers with damage to Broca's region (a portion of the brain located within the frontal region) were impaired of their capacity to make speech, and rarely recovered these skills. As research has revealed more connections between certain brain regions and their functions, the idea that we rely on certain brain regions for different cognitive functions becomes more common.

It has been over the last few years that we've observed the way the brain functions in real-time. Studies on animals and humans have demonstrated the brain's capacity to create new neural connections in response to events and deliberate thought patterns. Today, we have access to technologies that examine the connectivity between, as well as the functioning of specific neurons. We are able to scan both animal and human brains when they perform different cognitive tasks. Additionally, we can record pictures regularly which allows us to study the connection between behavior change and neuronal activity.

Neuroplasticity and its effects

A significant turning point in the field of neuroplasticity was the realization that individuals with brain injuries have the ability to recuperate the abilities they have lost. When an brain region that is usually is responsible for a particular task has been damaged proper training, another area of the brain may be able to take over. Furthermore, damaged areas of the brain are restored and eventually recovered if a suitable program of rehabilitation continues to be adhered to.

In the case of a person who is suffering from stroke (an occasion where blood clots prevent the flow of oxygen into the brain or to one or more within the brain) the patient will usually be left with issues with speaking or moving on the other part of the body. To allow the patient return to the ability to move their limbs and speech ability, they'll be required to adhere to an extensive rehabilitation program. The core of any structured recovery plan is a series of exercise that are repeated over the course of a few days months, weeks, and even years. The reasoning is easy for the purpose of helping damaged regions of the brain recover it is essential to stimulate new connections to form between neurons that are already in place and to promote neurogenesis. This way, neural networks that were previously inactive are reactivated, and patients will be able to regain the abilities they lost.

The study of healthy volunteers has demonstrated the fact that whenever we are deprived of our ability to see, other senses increase as a result. Researchers at the University of Montreal have shown that when we're removed from our sense of sight for just 90 minutes, we become more adept at being adept at detecting sound in the space. Additionally, those who are blind exhibit greater abilities in this regard than those who are visually impaired. This is further evidence to suggest that our brains are able to change quickly in response to different situations and external stimuli. Human brains have the remarkable ability of committing greater or lesser resources to certain functions based on the circumstances.

Why did our brains change to become plastic?

Humans are, without doubt, an extremely successful and developed species of Earth. Our ability to communicate complex thinking, intricate thought and the development of culture has allowed us to rule (for better or for worse) across the world. One of the major factors for this dominance is the way that our brains are able to adapt to any new challenge we encounter. This is why humans have been able to create an area of their own in nearly every type of environment. It doesn't matter if we're on a frozen tundra , or in tropical forests, every human community has found strategies to deal with the dangers and challenges that they face. Over the many tens thousands of years that have shaped the evolution of humans the ones who were the most adaptable to changing environments - i.e. the ones with the most flexible brains are the ones most likely to flourish in difficult environments, and then transfer this capability to their children.

How do taxi driver and musicians, as well as jugglers and taxi drivers have in the common?

Psychologists are also able to demonstrate neuroplasticity by using brain scanning techniques like Magnetic Resonance Imaging (known as MRI). The most renowned studies of neuroplasticity was a study that included London taxi driver. The process of becoming a driver in the capital city isn't easy and to be successful, you have to acquire a thorough understanding about the layout of London. This knowledge is referred to appropriately in the title "The Knowledge," and the test they have to pass to get their full license is called "The Knowledge Test." A typical wannabe driver must learn for years how navigate through the more than 25,000 roads that are within a 6-mile distance of Charing Cross at the heart of London.

This particular skill makes London taxi drivers a special case of further study. The researchers Eleanor Maguire and Katherine Woollett located in University College London, decided to study whether the process of studying "The Knowledge" left an impression, literally on the brains of drivers. They conducted brain scans on 79 new drivers over a period of years, employing MRI technology to observe the changes in their brains that were triggered by the intense course of studying. The process of studying for the test is so difficult that, in the end only 39 out of the 79 participants were able to pass the test. In the end, researchers were able to track the development of three groups: the ones who were trained to be taxi drivers who passed their test and those who had training but failed to pass as well as a control group of people who had never completed any training at all.

Their findings were amazing. In the driver trainees who were taught the city's layout and completed exams, the hippocampus, part of the brain that is responsible for spatial learning - increased in size. The same effect did not occur in the group of control or those who attempted to learn "The Knowledge" but later failed the test. Additionally, ongoing research shows that the longer someone has a job in the taxi industry the bigger their hippocampus gets. This is a fantastic illustration of how when you have the right mindset and focus you can actually mold your brain by being exposed to new ideas and experiences.

Musicians have also contributed to the study of neuroplasticity. A study that was published by the journal Frontiers in Psychology suggests that the practice of music alters the brain's structure and function. It's likely that brains of those who perform a musical instrument regularly improve their ability to combine auditory input as well as executing motor movements in response to stimulus. When you listen to the music or play an instrument simultaneously your brain is compelled to connect auditory and visual information. It is therefore likely that training in music encourages the process called "audio-visual integration." With more practice and dedication to playing an instrument your brain will get proficient at this form of processing.

The research has also examined the impact of short-term training on particular brain areas. For instance, a study released in PLoS One described a study that involved healthy adult volunteers who were taught how to play with balls. Twenty participants were taught how to juggle using three balls prior to having their brains tested seven 14, and 35 days after. After one few weeks of regular training the volunteers' Occipital lobes were altered. In particular, the region called V5 that is responsible for finding things in the air, a process essential for successful throwing and catching balls from juggling - was becoming more dense. This is a straightforward easy to understand illustration of the way that human brains change in direct response to effort and input. The study showed that for as long as participants continued to practice of juggling, these changes were maintained. However, when they stopped practicing the new skill, their occipital brain lobes returned to their pre-juggling condition. The findings of the study on juggling also suggest that learning a new skill even if it appears specific and niche, could prove beneficial in different scenarios. For example, if the ability to juggle improves your ability to quickly discern and identify objects in the space, so you can respond appropriately to them, it can improve your driving skills and make you a safer driver.

How can neuroplasticity affect your life?

Once you are aware of how flexible your brain can be and you begin to realize its potential to alter your life! Due to the brain's ability to change that allows you to acquire new abilities, and alter your outlook and attitude. Think about how much more productive you can achieve at work if changed your brain's wiring to improve focus, or how much happier you'd be if you trained your brain to have happier thoughts! The next chapters will show you how to enhance each aspect of your life with useful, simple exercises.

Establishing the foundations Diet and sleep

As you've already observed that your choices and actions are a key factor in the development of your brain and abilities. To ensure that your brain has the best opportunity to develop new neuronal networks, you must maintain the health of your body. It is therefore important to live your life as healthy as you can. Healthy brains are one that is healthy and a brain that is open to the new experience.

It is first and foremost essential to get enough rest. It's simple and straightforward, yet the majority of Western adults don't get the minimum of 6-8 hours a night that is recommended by the majority of health professionals. Although it's certain that some people require longer sleep hours than the others, the odds are that 8 hours of sleep per night is an ideal starting point. You could always cut down on the time you are in bed when you are able to function using less. It may seem to be a great strategy for maximising your time and accomplishing more however, it could result in a negative impact. Sleep deprivation can result in lower concentration levels as well as higher levels of stress hormones and a diminished concentration and have a harder time making choices.

Exercise: Schedule Your Sleep

Have a closer look at your bedroom. Is your bed comfortable? Are your bedrooms free of distractions? If you switch the lights off at the end of the night, is your bedroom sufficiently dark to ensure that you have a peaceful night's sleep? If you're finding it difficult to sleep in the evening, you can try making a routine for bed which helps you relax before bed. Based on your personal style and personal preferences, this could include activities like meditation (more about this in the text) and a relaxing bath or reading a few pages of a positive book, snuggling with pets or a loved one or keeping a journal or taking a moment to reflect on what you enjoyed about the day.

Diet is a crucial factor when trying to improve your brain's function. In order to ensure healthy connections between neurons your body requires an ongoing supply of omega-3 fats. These are present in soybeans, oily fish and walnuts, flaxseeds and flaxseeds as well as spinach , and chia seeds. Try eating 3-4 pieces of fish oily, such as mackerel every week, and then add the other food items listed above as frequently as possible.

Antioxidants are essential in keeping the brain healthy. They are typically found in vegetables and fruits. They are beneficial for the brain as they protect it from oxidative stress, an organic reaction that takes place as a result of your cells interfacing with oxygen, and then releasing molecules called "free radicals" which can cause cell damage. Oxidative stress is also consequence of the interaction of pollution and harmful chemicals such as alcohol, smoking and air pollution being the main factors. It is good to know that antioxidants can help reduce the effects of this issue. It is recommended to consume at least five portions of fruits and vegetables each day. These should be eaten raw or steamed, not boiled or fried, since extreme cooking techniques can significantly reduce the antioxidant amount.

Exercise: Make A Brain Food Shopping List
Take a look at what you consume during the course of your day. Are you getting sufficient omega-3 fats as well as antioxidants? In the event that you don't, what do you include them in your diet frequently? Simple modifications like adding berries to your breakfast cereal, or substituting red meat with oily fish on a night of the week can be a big help in preserving the neuroplasticity of your brain.

Chapter 14: Guide To Increase Your Neuroplasticity And Development Encounters

You are able to create new neural pathways up to the day you drop the bucket.

What is the reason this change the situation?

As with any other muscles that you have in your body, it is either utilize it or you lose it. Thus, keeping your mind drawn into and continuously reworking it is essential for your continued intellectual performance as well as your general well-being.

Neuroplasticity, also known as cerebrum plancy is the capacity of your brain to reorganize itself in your behavior, condition thoughts, and emotions. You are able to do this physically and mentally for all of your life.

Before the time that Dr. Norman Doidge, a specialist at University of Toronto University of Toronto, inquired about the benefits of neuroplasticity widely believed that cerebrums were a fixed organ that could not be changed. Today, we know that cerebrum flexibility is a fluid phenomenon and has been utilized to benefit, helping combat conditions such as various sclerosis, stroke, Parkinson's disease and mental imbalance and many more.

From the myth of ageing #7: the way of aging isn't dependent on your personal qualities. 75percent of way that you age is within your control and your personal circumstances as well as your lifestyle and behavior are more likely to have an influence on the way you reach your age than the 25% of your age attributed to your talents.

Tips: Your behavior matters when it comes to working your brain. Therefore, making every day a miniaturized movement to break free of negative habits is essential to a successful maturation.

Where is it that it occurs?

As per Linda Overstreet-Wadiche, a specialist as well as Jacques Wadiche at the University of Alabama at Birmingham

Department of Neurobiology There are two important cerebrum locations that are constantly producing new neurons, even in adults.

Hippocampus is your central point for long-distance and spatial memory

Cerebellum, your center point for coordination and memory of muscles

The four components of your brain are responsible for the majority of your memories with the hippocampus and cerebellum are the two regions that have the highest rate of neurogenesis.

The reason behind the reason these two regions of your mind are crucial for neuroplasticity is due to the fact that they're filled with granule cells neurons, which exhibit the highest rate of neurogenesis.

There was a well-known study conducted on the neuroplasticity of London taxi drivers as well as transport drivers. Transport drivers had significantly smaller hippocampuses when they drove on the same route regularly as taxi drivers, who depended on their cerebrums to continuously be able to explore various day by day course.

What can we do to be proactive?

When you are immersed in exciting inspiring, stimulating and exciting experiences you'll be able to take part in intense challenges that can be used as an element of your ongoing learning. To help you do this, I've put together this guide bit-by-bit on the most efficient method of building your neuroplasticity as well as develop your experiences.

Step 1: Identify lucidity

Enhancing your brain's versatility is a matter of altering your habits. Additionally, prior to embarking for any major change in your behavior Many people do not grasp the fundamental step of finding clarity. Knowing exactly what you must to accomplish and even crucial reasons you have to do it, is essential for implementing genuine changes as long as is possible.

The process of determining what's at the heart of your worth-based framework is huge. Your primary principle along with your desires and personal characteristics all play the primary role of guiding your activities and providing you with a true belief in the importance of your actions and the rationale behind them.

If you're happy and sharing the things that matter to you, you'll be able to continue your positive methods that test you and assist you in developing over years of... good constructive criticism circles.

Once you have a clear understanding of your fundamental beliefs, you are able to begin to reorient everything else around the guiding principles. This arrangement of your primary beliefs is crucial to making more conscious decisions, which in turn helps your brain expand.

Step #2: Set important goals

If you're clear you'll be able to concentrate on the most important goals you'll be able to establish for yourself, as well as an understanding of what goals to tackle first. Setting objectives is crucial in preparing yourself for a lifetime of learning and it is an essential part of enhancing your neuroplasticity.

TIP: Consider thinking beyond the complexities of cerebrum games and riddles. To truly draw your brain to the maximum extent possible take a look at more significant experiences which will test your mind and stimulate your curiosity.

Reward Tip: If it's possible to take part in activities and goals that work on the engine, visual and sound components of your brain This is a full body mind-training exercise that requires you to be connected with you corpus callosum. This will build the spanned relationships between your left brain and right cerebrum. That will enable you to be more adept at handling complex issues and will have better coordination.

For help in setting important objectives for your life, evaluate your energy level in the four classes in these centers. Find out which part of your life you're in and what you would like to be in all of these aspects that make up your day-to-day life

Your Network is your personal social network at the local level regardless of whether they're your family members, friends neighbors, partners, neighbors or even strangers Social communication is crucial to your health and general success.

Development - experiences, people and activities that test you. A few questions to think about: How could you develop an impactful and stimulating knowledge available to yourself? What have you been fascinated by? What goals would you like to accomplish with the aim of having no doubts about life? What has it been that you've needed to secure an expectation chest due to life's events that has disrupted your normal flow?

Giving back - irrespective of whether you're making an estate donation, or giving your time and talents Giving back is beneficial for your mental, energetic and physical well-being. Volunteerism can satisfy your desire to be necessary and give you an underlying sense of direction whether you're offering help to your neighbors and family members.

Wellbeing is a matter of working out and eating right as well as your mental and physical wellbeing. Where are the best practices on your priority list?

From these four central categories for maturing successfully complete the associated activity:

Imagine your life in the present.

What do you wish to make different about this part that you live in?

What are your bad habits?

What are the best habits you are?

Select from the 4 central classes to be focused on and then use the subject to create your initial goal. Then, you'll be able to create a goal specific to you which then becomes an opening for you to expand your mind with to be able to attain that particular goal.

Here are a few more conceptual questions to help you to focus the scope of a particular goal:

What would you be able to do if you had more confidence and no fear that could impede the traffic?

Have you ever required to know?

What else do you want to be involved in and accomplish so that you don't have second thoughts?

What are the things you've needed to keep an expectation chest, because life interrupted your routine?

To make it easier, make your goal an SMART target and ensure that it is precise, but also quantifiable, achievable appropriate, and reasonable.

You're now ready to take a step.

Step 3: Take small steps

Do your best to take the maximum tiny steps every single day while you are moving towards your goal. One of the things you must avoid is overwhelm yourself with an too much to accomplish or, even more incredibly the overly large target that leaves you not knowing where to start.

To help you set up small-scale projects to reach your goals, you should initially be able to think the vast array of ideas that you could do to get there. The more ideas you come up with and the more imaginative your ideas will become.

134

From there you will not only have plenty of ideas to write down on paper, but your brain will begin to imagine and think ingenuously especially as you plan your goal.

It's amazing how you can completely and logically concentrate at the details of... it's amazing what happens when you focus on process is revealed.

You could also keep a daily journal or log, where you write down a simple task that you complete each day to increase your progress toward your goal. You must push yourself to improve your performance consistently. If you are able to incorporate this into your daily routine it's where you'll most likely discover your superpower.

What's the reason? By focussing on small pieces of development at once and you'll become more cultivated in your confidence, more assured and more able to try again. According to an Harvard Business Review article, the importance of small success lies in the improvement of the standard:

"Of the considerable number of things that can help feelings, inspiration, and observations during a workday, the absolute most significant is gaining ground in important work."

Tip: Be predictable. It's better to set smaller daily goals than to have an ambitious goal less often. If you're having trouble keeping up, break your day-to-day activities task into something smaller.

When your brain first starts recording changes, the underlying changes to your cerebrum are not permanent. In order to make lasting enhancements to your cerebrum's design and to build the best mind-splitting abilities, you need to be on the lookout for ways to test your brain every day.

Step #4: Adopt a development attitude

The development mindset step is the most fundamental one and allows you to to tap into your feelings of endurance and strength. Song Dweck's study did a good amount of the exam chipping away at establishing an outlook for development based of "the possibility that we can develop our cerebrum's ability to learn and to take care of issues."

The main reason to build an attitude of development is that it is a part of overcoming the difficulties.

When you're pursuing any goal or test using a growth mindset be sure to look at the potential traps and prepare for "disappointments" or agony focuses as being buried in the difficult moments and unpleasant encounters can be a great source of growth and learning. The majority of us have anxieties, and we keep the distance from problems due to our fears of anxiety, but should you be able to aim directly at the issues and locate them it will make a massive difference.

Three increasingly significant tips on the development of a mindset:

Pay attention to the steps

Find a valuable analysis

Don't look for endorsements

Tips: To truly have an attitude of development that prepares you for a lifetime of learning, set an additional goal for every objective you accomplish. This allows you to focus more on making the most out of the process as well as the journey itself.

Step #5: Practice care

Mindfulness is such a ground-breaking concept in the development of any new (and excellent) behavior. When you're more conscious of your surroundings and your thoughts and are more aware of what's going on within your brain and your awareness it's likely that you'll choose based on worth which are fundamentally superior and more important decisions.

It's linked to the following:

Mindfulness

Refrain from settling on worth decisions based on worth

The root of the majority of our bad habits are poor habits and bad decisions. In addition, a substantial part of them are subconscious which we do not ever think about. According to an Roberts Wesleyan College article, we are able to make 35,000 decisions each day.

In the pursuit of this goal, we make a few poor decisions based on esteem every day.

According to an investigation written by experts Bas Verplanken as well as Rob Holland:

People take decisions in line to their personal characteristics, only in case those traits are triggered psychologically.

In terms of expanding your neuroplasticity, and changing the brain's experiences it is crucial. If you're a slave to autopilot (which most of us do) It will likely require extra energy to get used to awakening your prefrontal cortex. It's the most fundamental part of your brain, before creating any new habit.

It's an essential element of increasing your awareness, and you'll be equipped to apply your judgment and to fill your day with things that matter to you.

Here are a few ideas regarding rehearsing the care of children:

Write down your thoughts in a journal and reflect on the things you're grateful for.

Establish a solid morning routine

Do breathing exercises or reflect on your breathing.

Practice yoga, judo or chi gong

Connect to nature

Concentrate on the agenda of activities

Detox from the internet-based life and media

Spend less money on advanced devices and spend less time watching TV

Focus on your vision the core beliefs, goals and list

Tips: Work through your thoughts. According to Neuroscientist Wendy Suzuki: "Thinking quickly changes the recurrence of your cerebrum waves and, following five years, builds the size of white issue packages in the prefrontal cortex."

Warning: You could create bad habits in your day by merely. This is another reason to pay attention to what's happening upstairs , and to keep track of your ideas for designs.

Being a person who lives each day with expectations especially when you decide to set your pace on a daily schedule, will be more likely to influence your actions and choices throughout the day.

Step #6: Carefully choose the hover of your the impact

Your ability to make an impact is so impressive. You are the person you spend your energy with So, take advantage of it.

Tips: Let those who share your basic beliefs to join your circle of concern and decrease the number of people who are not in your circle of influence.

If you spend more time with people who share your fundamental beliefs It is likely that you will have significant experiences of development which will increase your neuroplasticity.

Begin to surround yourself with people who can help you focus on your progress goals, health and qualities, as well as the reason. The more time you spend with the right people and exercise, the more likely you will experience a greater sense of energy and activating the fundamental leadership portion of your brain.

The importance of social interaction especially among older people is crucial in terms of your health - both truly and physically. If you adapt your networks of buddies to your personal characteristics and goals for development This could be the most powerful formula to improve your cerebrum health.

Step 7: Prioritize your schedule of activities

A recent study conducted by Kirk Erickson and associates that linked "more noteworthy measures of physical action to less cortical decay, better mind work and improved intellectual capacity."

The group also discovered that:

"Physical action exploits the cerebrum's characteristic limit with regards to versatility."

If it's an extreme and vigorous anaerobic exercise or light and active exercise that is supported, try to integrate in your day to day schedule some kind of exercise timetable. Here are some suggestions of oxygen-consuming activities you to consider:

Good preparation: lift loads to the vast most of your muscular groups at a minimum, two unsuccessful days in a row. It is possible to begin with light and easy and gradually add more sets and weights each week. Be sure to warm your body first prior to lifting.

Cardio - walking or biking, swimming and tennis or climbing. Begin small and work to increase your frequency and time each week. A good starting point is 10 minutes 3 days per week, and then stir it up until you're able to do 30 minutes five times every week. Be sure to get warm and stretch later.

Balance becomes more important as we get older. Try to incorporate the practices of extending and adaptability with your regular routine, such as yoga, kendo, or chi gong. Other ways to achieve equalization include using activities balls, walking with an e-book on your head or laying on your back for as long as you are able and even while your eyes are closed in case you're taking the test.

Tip: Connect with nature. This is a fantastic way to beat out the two stages of #5 and #7. If you're outdoors, it could boost the transient memory of 20% according to an experiment conducted by University of Michigan. University of Michigan.

Step #8: Stop hesitating

The more you repress the need to alter your behavior and habits more difficult it will be to develop your mind's flexibility. Furthermore, if you stop dragging, your mind is more likely to letting go of the use the rule of "lose it.

The 19 tips from 19 Tips for a Wonderful Retirement, here are two methods to help your move quickly. You can move using two of my favorite strategies that actually work:

Mel Robbins' 5 Second Rule - when you sense the need to make an objectively based decision then you count in reverse 5-4-3-2-1, and then physically move to make the move. The theory behind how this method works is:

"If you have a motivation to follow up on an objective, you should physically move inside 5 seconds or your mind will kill the thought."

Dwindle Voogd's Deliberation Train is that you don't wait up until you are ready to do something. Instead, you perform some pre-planning and make your decision first, and then later and finally feel. Many people fail to make an action because they perform opposite and first feel before making their decisions.

Both theories are based on the assumption that if you stall until you're ready to do something, you're not going to be able to complete it because you're not going to think about it. Therefore, a way to get rid of dawdling is to trick your brain into moving in the fastest way possible before the brain gets a grip on everything.

It is possible to prepare your mind to begin making quick decisions.

Step #9: Raise your benchmarks

Tony Robbins put it compactly:

"If you need to change your life you need to increase your expectations."

Being proactive and taking preventive steps to prepare for your own aging You're in the process of increasing your expectations. You're transforming our way of living in order to avoid the age-related effects by taking care of your future self and creating the example for those who follow, so be grateful for doing just about everything.

Prakhar Verma published an article that was published in an article published on The Mission:

"You increase your expectations each time when you - disregard the reptile cerebrum, say no to interruptions, postpone gratification or pick intentional uneasiness."

To ensure that you are in good fitness, always keep your own responsibility and follow these nine steps consistently and with a lot of effort. By keeping your objectives and progress at the forefront edge of your thinking You'll be drowned in achieving your objectives, but also effectively stimulating your brain to use the right muscles to maintain your vision.

Chapter 15: Mind And Body

We imagine our bodies and our minds as separate entities, yet they are directly impacted by one another. Your thoughts affect the way your body functions and the reverse is true. The more you can collaborate with your entire body the easier it will be for you to achieve the best brain you can get.

Stomach-Brain Relationship

When we get ready for our stomachs, it is common to consider food. The stomach is where we go to process the food we consume. There's also a wealth of new information on the relationship with your gut and brain.

What we aren't aware of often is the amount of hormones that are released inside the intestines of your body. Have you ever noticed something going on in the stomach while you were feeling anxious or anxious?

Do you frequently experience stomach pains after day of stress?

Of of course, the food you consume can have a profound impact on the way you think. In reality it's the hormones that are produced that influence our brain. The mere thought of eating can alter the chemical signals released by the stomach.

If you experience constant stomach pains, heartburn or any other digestive issues It could be due to anxiety. If you experienced stomach ache, the initial thought you'll have is that something was wrong with what you ate. However, it could be something that is happening in your brain.

It is time to listen to our stomachs in the same way we do our brains. This is the reason why it's not a bad idea to tell yourself, "Go with your gut." It's possible that you need to listen to your stomach at least once every so often.

In order for your brain to perform to its maximum potential It is important to think about the way that our food choices influence the hormones produced in our stomachs. The stomach is in fact a microbiome. This means that there are microbes in your stomach responsible for breaking down food items by transferring various minerals and vitamins to various parts of your body.

If you're not taking care of your stomach correctly and only filling it with acidic food items, fats that are difficult to digest, as well as white carbohydrates, which could be a challenge for your stomach too. This can be seen in your brain. People who consume unhealthy foods frequently may find that they are suffering from serious issues regarding your mental wellbeing. Let's examine another thing that could be detrimental for your body: inflammation.

The Dangers of Inflammation

Think about the last time mosquitos was a biting victim to you.

The first thing you could be feeling is some discomfort or itching in your face. Following this, you may have a tiny bump of red.

Consider the time you scrape or cut yourself. The first cut is in which the skin was ripped open. Around it, it gets thick and red. The reason is inflammation.

Inflammation is the body's defense mechanism to protect itself from potentially harmful external sources. White blood cells, as well as other forms of attack are triggered when there's an external source which could cause dangerous infections. The body has this natural reaction to shield yourself from things which could be damaging to your body. There is a lot of inflammation that we notice on the outside of our bodies. However, what we aren't aware of is that it can happen also on the inside.

If you're eating chemicals and other harmful substances it could result in inflammation of the brain. Since the brain is the first organ to receive the nutrients it needs from whatever you consume in order to ensure that it is fueled with enough energy this indicates the brain has been utilizing chemicals, additives, and other toxic sources to fuel its needs. This can cause inflammation in the brain, meaning it's not working as well or perform as well as it might.

To make sure the level of inflammation is in control, it is important to take a look at the additives are in our diet and the ingredients will help fight inflammation and help our bodies in the long run. Let's look at the worst foods your brain could be exposed to, and the top foods that you ought to include more of.

Worst Foods for Your Brain

One of the most harmful foods that can harm the brain are sugar. Sugar is essential for survival. The sugar is present in blood and is how we handle the various substances we consume. But, sugar added to our diets can be dangerous. Sugar is present in everyday items such as baked items, soda, sweets and other extremely sweet foods.

Sugar is also present in a variety of ingredients, including white pasta and bread.

We add sugar and many other items to make it taste better. Sugar is also extremely addictive. It's not just that sugar can have negative effects on the body, but a addiction to sugar can make you feel tired, grumpy and lead to difficulty in concentration and fatigue.

Sugar is present in refined carbohydrates which are carbs which are processed. Think of bread, grains pasta, bread, and the similar to that, while the week is always the best choice. When you next visit the supermarket, make sure you choose whole wheat pasta, bread as well as other carbs items like brown rice or quinoa are the best choices.

Anything that has been processed is also likely to have lots of additives. Salt and other chemicals are added in food items to help the food last for longer. Fresh and whole grain does not keep as long which is why lots of people prefer buying processed foodsthat are less expensive and last longer than fresh food items. However, they often end up buying unhealthful food.

It's easy to consume in a variety of ways, and then processed.

Additionally, it contains a lot of other additives, such as food dyes and chemicals that allow it to last for longer. They are good for your brain and may directly contribute to an increase in inflammation levels, think about other ingredients that aren't just connected with healthy food also.

There are additives that are found in foods with no sugar, like diet soda that can cause inflammation. These substances make foods taste sweet and sweet without sugar added, but the substance itself can be equally damaging for your brain. Although you may not gain weight the way you do when eating normal sweetened foods with added sugar but you may be able to experience negative impacts on your cognitive abilities.

It is also important to reduce our consumption of alcohol. Certain alcohols may cause you to feel more relaxed, but there are elements in these drinks that can trigger detrimental effects to the brain. It's the excess of these, and is the most harmful. If you indulge in sweets here there, drink the occasional diet soda after dinner, have a glass of wine or eat a greasy fast food restaurant, it's okay every once in a period of time. If you do these activities daily, it can create inflammation. It won't be noticeable immediately however you'll feel the effects and your brain won't perform as well that it can. To focus on improving the neuroplasticity your brain, be sure not to consume too much of these food items. Instead, let's consider some delicious foods you can consume instead of these items (Mandi 2018.).

Best Brain Power Foods

The best foods to eat is omega-3 acid fatty acids.

They help ensure that the brain cells in your body are steady; they make healthy neurons and shield against any harm. Omega-3 fatty acids may also boost your circulation, and may aid in regulating inflammation. The best food source of omega-three fatty acids is healthy, fatty fish. They include tuna, salmon herring, sardines and mackerel.

It is also possible to consume anti-inflammatory food items such as berries or spinach, right away. They're loaded with antioxidants. Antioxidants are crucial and can help to fight inflammation.

Choose dark berries like blackberries, blueberries, and raspberries. Pick green leafy spinach and eat them raw to reap the highest amount of antioxidants. A lot of people prefer to add them in smoothies too as it is a fantastic option to eat spinach as well as other greens that are leafy because it reduces it to in a way that is as minimal as it can be. It is possible to mask them in smoothies , too and make use of things like sweet berries and honey to disguise the flavor. It's a fantastic method to increase the amount of inflammation you're absorbing.

Furthermore take into consideration whole grains. As we said earlier ensure that whatever you purchase doesn't simply state the ingredients. It should be 100% whole wheat. You may also have drinking a glass of red wine every now and then or a slice (or two) of dark chocolate. Both of them contain anti-inflammatory properties and will help you achieve optimal brain functioning and also (Burgess 2018, 2018).

The Importance of Physical Exercise

Healthy eating is vital however, we must also to make sure we're getting enough of physical activity.

There is no need for everyone to purchase an account at a gym and train for hours every day. What you should ensure is that you're taking regular walks and dancing, doing lighter weight lifting and participating in activities which will get you moving. Make sure you're doing what's comfortable for your body. Find something that can be done with friends Make it a social event so that you're not so easily distracted. Listen to music and have a blast. Find a group of friends to play baseball or visit the local park to play basketball. If you're in your 40s, 30s or 50s does not mean you cannot be able to visit the park and play with your pals. Whatever you decide to do, you should look for ways to alleviate your anxiety instead of making new stressors.

Mindfulness and Meditation

You can consume the most nutritious food items in the world, be the most athletic individual you've ever met and also be one of the crazy health nuts you've seen on fitness ads.

If your life isn't managing the anxiety at the end of the day, all of this won't be as important. Stress can cause heart attacks, even if you haven't consumed a single ounce of fat over the last 10 years.

Stress can cause damage to your body. One of the most effective ways to deal with stress is to practice meditation and mindfulness. These are simple practices that don't require fitness membership, a nutritionist or anything else to ease anxiety. We'll start by focusing on mindfulness. Mindfulness is the method of focusing on the present when you're feeling anxious. It's possible that you're worried about the future or you may be too focussed on the past. To be aware it is important to focus yourself present in the moment.

An easy act of mindfulness is looking at your surroundings and paying attention to the people around you. For a better understanding focus on one thing, choose one to concentrate on. For instance, now go through the room and notice things made of wood. Have you tried this? That's mindfulness! This is all it requires. Let's try it again. Check out the room and note everything with the color green.

How did that go? This is also an aspect of mindfulness. It is also possible to engage your senses. You can identify a scent you detect. Look for something is a sound. What can you feel? What are you able to taste? What do you be able to see? It's all mindfulness, because it draws your attention from where it was , and brings it to the present moment.

The practice of meditation is an intense kind of mindfulness. It is the practice of taking a particular part of your day and focusing your attention on nothing in particular. It is a chance to relax completely and discover peace in your mind to completely let the thoughts go from your mind. Begin with guided meditation exercises to give you a clear understanding of what this process involves.

Chapter 16: Understanding

Regenerative Medicine

The body is naturally capable to heal itself. It has its own process which repair damaged cells. There is an ongoing process of replacing damaged cells in order to keep tissues in good condition. If tissues are damaged cells begin to limit the damage and then begin replacing the damaged cells. Consider skin wounds as a case in point. Body heals, and new cells are created over the wound.

Regenerative medicine takes those inherent ability and enhances it. This field is designed to help the body to improve self-healing mechanisms and take it further. Regenerative medicine aim to accelerate healing, and also rebuild the normal structure and functioning of injured tissues. They will be used to treat diseases which conventional medicine has declared incurable.

Consider Alzheimer's disease, ALS and similar degenerative diseases. The current treatments are only effective in slowing the process. It's not working in the majority of patients. The diseases are getting worse, which medicine cannot stop it.

It's also the case for permanent damaged tissues. A lot of people live with organs that are considered permanently damaged. They may suffer permanent damage to their reproductive organs because of radiation exposure or due to an illness. It could result in permanently damaged nerves due to an accident. It could be permanent damage to brain cells that have been damaged by trauma to the brain.

Modern medicine might appear to have advanced exponentially in the last few decades, however there are huge limitations on how it is able to heal.

Restorative medicine is a way to treat irreparably damaged organs and treatable ailments. The field is based on four basic concepts.

Medical devices and artificial organs are becoming useful in many medical conditions. Regenerative medicine is a method of improving the quality of life by developing technology that allows people to maintain a good health despite being affected by illnesses. For instance, regenerative medicine has recently created artificial organs that allow people to have a healthier and more fulfilling life, despite having spina Bifida. Regenerative medicine created technology to assist these patients in having more control over their bladders.

Regenerative medicine also concentrates on biomaterials and tissue engineering. One of the primary objectives in this area is to help humans to eventually remove the necessity of replacing entire organs that are hurt or destroyed. Biomaterials and tissue repair can aid the body in its ability to recover and restore normal function, without needing the need to repair damaged organs by artificial ones.

For instance, those suffering from severe heart issues such as those with a damaged heart valves are limited to having a heart transplantation as their only alternative. Heart valves damaged or defective are replaced by mechanical devices. They can help, but they are not as efficient or durable in comparison to the initial heart valve tissue.

Regenerative medicine investigates the possibility of developing the human heart valves the laboratory. They are less risky in comparison to existing options.

The tissues will come from patients' own tissue. This will significantly decrease the possibility of rejection.

Clinical trials have proved very successful in this aspect. The trials are extremely promising, and it shouldn't take long before these will be available to the general population.

Heart valves are only the beginning. Regenerative medicine is aiming to address more demands in the medical area. This involves regenerating more complicated body parts, including the entire kidneys, heart and not just the smaller tissues. This could be further developed , and the same technology could be utilized to create whole limbs for amputees.

Cellular therapies can be a innovative treatments for various diseases. There are many options to utilize cell therapy. The new cells replace the damaged ones. These cells could originate from healthy organs within the body of the patient. Many may choose their cells stored in cryoporation for later use when they are required. For instance the blood cells of the umbilical cord of a baby could be stored to treat cellular diseases later throughout the life of the child.

There are many medical advantages. A child who is born with the genes for a specific disease could utilize those blood vessels from their umbilical cord to aid in treatment.

This kind of treatment is more commonly referred to as stem therapy using cells. It is a broad field of application that have the biggest effect on the treatment of degenerative conditions like cancer or severe brain injury or injuries to the spinal cord caused by traumatic injuries. It is also used to improve health overall or counteract the consequences of the aging process. As an example stem cells can be utilized to replace cells found in joints and muscles that have been affected by arthritis. Stem cells can also be utilized to treat specific types of cancers, including leukemia. A few are also beginning to use stem cells to aid in the treatment of infertility.

Many are making use of it for aesthetic reasons for example, replacing wrinkled, sagging skin using stem cells to promote healthier, younger skin.

This is one of the areas that Regenerative medicine is currently focusing specifically on its contribution for helping the body return to the normal structure and attain the highest level of functioning.

The translation of clinical research is an important aspect of the field of regenerative medicine.

Chapter 17: Limited Set Of Routes

For a long time it was thought that as we grew older as we grew older, connections in our brain became stale but then they faded. Research has proven that the brain never ceases to change as it learns. Plasticity refers to the capacity that the brain has to adapt as it learns.

The changes that occur as a result of learning happen typically at the level connections between neurons. connections develop and the structure and internals of existing synapses changes. Do you realize that once you are a pro in a particular area that the parts of your brain that are involved in the skills you've acquired will increase?

For example, London taxi drivers have an hippocampus that is larger (in the area of the posterior) in comparison to London bus driver. Why is this? It's because this part of the hippocampus has been specialized in processing and storing intricate spatial information to effectively navigate. Taxi drivers are required to navigate through London and bus drivers must follow only a few routes.

The same phenomenon can be observed within the brains of people who are bilingual. It appears that the ability to learn the second language is achievable by undergoing functional changes in the brain. For instance, the left superior parietal cortex appears to be bigger in brains of bilinguals than monolingual brains.

There are also changes in the plasticity of musicians ' brains when compared with non-musicians. Gaser and Schlaug studied the brains of professional musicians (who perform at least an hour each day) to amateur musicians as well as non-musicians. They discovered the gray matter (cortex) volume was the highest among professional musicians. It was moderate for the amateur musician, and at its lowest for non-musicians in a variety of brain regions that are that are involved in music playing including motor regions, the anterior superior parietal regions, and the inferior temporal area.

Then, Draganski and colleagues recently discovered that the intensive learning of abstract concepts can cause some changes in the brain. They examined the cerebral cortexes of German medical students three months before the medical exam and immediately following the test, and compared them with brains of students who weren't taking exams at the moment. Medical students' brains revealed changes induced by learning in the regions that are part of the cortex parietal aswell in the hippocampus posterior. These brain regions are thought to be involved in learning and memory retrieval.

The brain and its plasticity

The most interesting aspect of neuroplasticity is that brain activity that is associated with a specific function may actually shift to a new location because of experiences or brain injury.

The book " The Brain That Changes Itself: Stories of Personal Triumph from the Frontiers of Brain Science," Norman Doidge describes numerous instances of functional shifts. In one the story, the surgeon in his 50s is struck by an injury called a stroke. He is left disabled. As he recovers the hand and arm are restricted and he's set to wash tables. It's initially difficult. Slowly, the arm that is injured learns to move. He is able to write again, and to play tennis again. The functions of the brain regions that were damaged by the stroke are transferred into healthy brain regions!

The brain compensates for damaged by reorganizing itself and creating new connections between neurons that are intact. To reconnect, neurons need to be stimulated by activities.

Let me conclude by addressing two concerns we frequently get...

If you've ever set goals and hopes that didn't materialize You're not alone. A staggering ninety-two percent of those claim that their resolutions and goals are not met. they set themselves each year aren't achieving their goals.

Here are seven ideas for changing your thinking:

year never get achieved. With such high numbers it is something common that is preventing them from achieving their goals.

After reviewing the 8% that achieve the goals I've got some insights into the things that these top performers differ from the rest of us.

It is important to remember that the 8% of them come from every walk of life. They could be single, married or divorced, highly trained or even high school dropouts wealthy, middle class, or even poor according to the majority of norms. They're made up of various ethnicities and ages from across the globe.

The truth is that, regardless of where you are in your life or where you come from, you're equipped with the capability to set ambitious goals and reach them.

The main thing they share with people in the top 8 percent of people is the similar set of positive attitudes which guide their thoughts and actions. There are many of them but you may also be implementing opposite mental models without realizing that you are doing it.

One surefire method to determine whether you require to get a mental health check-up is to consider this question: Are you consistently achieving your objectives and living your dream? If you said "yes," read on and you'll be able to see the reason. If you answered "no," these steps could have a major impact on your life.

Here are seven ideas for how you can change your mental outlook:

1. Accept that your thinking requires adjustment It's normal to have hopes and goals that didn't go as we had hoped or envisioned. If this happens often and we begin to think about what needs to be changed. We rarely examine our own thoughts as a place to start making the necessary changes.

We live in a skill-based society that focuses on the development of new skills as well as improving the ones we're lacking. This is often a way of promoting the idea that we should be educated to reach our objectives. Some go back to school, while others attend classes and workshops, or go through books, constantly looking for the perfect skill set that can help everything come together.

I'm not saying that you shouldn't, I'm not denying the importance of knowledge and skills; however, most often, it's our mental models which require adjustments.

The best part is, it's much less costly and much quicker to alter your mental outlook than to learn new skills. Therefore, the first step is to accept that you'll need to focus on your mental state first.

2. Find your counter-mindsets Mindsets are developed through previous experiences and emotional milestones. The ones that don't yield the desired results are referred to as counter-mindsets.

A few examples are self-doubt and limiting beliefs or any of the other thoughts you have that can get out of the way of happiness.

A total of 65,000 thoughts are circulating our minds every day. In the majority of cases most of them are negative. The "Automatic Negative Thoughts" (ANTs) are so frequent that you're not conscious that they exist (most of us don't).

For instance: Do you know the voice in your head that screams out reckless spending habits while you're looking over your budget for the month? Or even makes negative comments when you glance at yourself in the mirror?

We've all heard that voice. It makes you hesitate prior to meeting someone you'd like meet. It causes you to consider rethinking your decision before launching an enterprise or contemplating changing careers.

Every person has different desires, and in the dark we're letting them to derail our hopes. It's difficult to stay optimistic when that voice keeps on ranting and saying things like "I can't talk to her," "I'm not smart enough," "I'm out of shape," "I'm not qualified" "... yada and you get the picture.

The best way to eliminate the ANTs within your head is to start paying close attention to the ant population. Pay attention to the dissident voice, and notice the frequency with which it occurs. Most likely, you'll discover that your ideas can be reduced to a handful of key issues. Making note of this is an important move because we are unable to change what we've not acknowledged.

3. Switch off the light - Once you've identified the top negative thoughts, it's time to find an effective method to prevent them from hindering your progress. The best method I've come across to do this is what I refer to as "flip the switch," that shifts the thoughts of negative thoughts to positive.

Over the years, each time I was in the mirror only what I saw was my shortcomings. Then, I began to practice exactly the opposite reaction, turning the switch. I would look at the mirror and try to think, "You look good!"

It took me a while to adjust with it. But the fact is that positive and negative thoughts don't share the same space, which is why I had to give my ANTs an expulsion notice.

Another approach I've found to be successful is known as"the "if/then" approach. Once you have identified the times when your ANTs usually appear, you can apply an idea process which allows you to imagine yourself out of them.

Let's take an example: you've planned to take an outing after dinner to increase your exercise however, after dinner you notice that your ANT is kicking in. If you begin to be able to hear that voice inside your head saying you're tired, or over-stuffed, or that you'll never shed the weight, then go into the closet to put on running sneakers.

In most cases, one step towards the right direction can be enough to put those ants up. Make an outline of if/then statements in advance.

4. Know what is your "why" Changing your mindsets requires effort because habits that have been formed aren't always easy to break. This is particularly true because many of our worst behaviors and mental states were formed as children, and we've

continued to behave exactly the same way since then.

Finding the importance of your "why" is about starting new and setting a objective or goal that, if you can achieve it, will result in the beginning of a new era. Losing weight. Finding yourself more content at work. Enhancing the relationship you have with your spouse. Look for something that could have an enormous difference on your life.

If it's going to require effort to bring it into reality It must be important, isn't it?

Once you know the "why" is, write down on paper or in a journal what it is that matters to you. It's not on a computer... in a notebook with your personal handwriting. This is an essential aspect of establishing your motivation.

5. Recognize that willpower and motivation aren't enough - Many people believe that willpower and motivation are all they need to accomplish their goals. It's no wonder that they do as it's the most typical advice you hear from your family

and friends to motivational gurus and coaches.

I suggested that you note down your main "why" in step four because that's the place where motivation kicks in. However, we all are aware that motivation is difficult to sustain, regardless of the importance of your goal be. This is when the willpower required to begin to kick in.

The most recent brain research has revealed that willpower functions as the capacity of a gasoline tank. It starts with a full tank, but you exhaust your tank every time you utilize it. This is what I mean by

You're trying to be healthier and then you go to work and discover Girl Scout cookies next to the fruit bowl. What can you do? Use your willpower to refuse to eat the cookies. Bravo!

You plan to exercise after work, but you end in staying late to handle an issue with a customer. You're already exhausted and the added pressure of not adhering to the original plan isn't helping.

Do you find yourself going to the fitness center? It's a given since it's happened every one of us.

It's not difficult to surrender and give up on our goals if we rely on determination and motivation to reach them. But they're not always enough. This is why 25 percent of people give up in the first week and 60% give up within one month.

High-achieving people understand this fact and that's the reason step five is about acknowledging... which is acknowledging that success isn't just about slapping your hands on the path to success.

If you accept this truth and letting it go, you'll stop blaming yourself for not sticking to your goals. This will leave you more energized and ready to take another shot tomorrow! (We'll go into more detail about this in step 7.)

6. Begin small, so that you can end up with a big goal - This may be counterintuitive, however one of the most effective ways to shift your perspective and achieve your goals is by setting outrageously small and utterly feasible objectives.

How small?

What about this: just one push-up.

If your main objective is to do regular exercising, the smaller but achievable objective is to complete just one push-up per day.

If you're looking to lessen the tension in your lifestyle, your nitty-gritty target could be to sit for a minute at evening.

If you're looking to have more love with your loved ones Your goal could be just one more embrace or kiss.

Each of these scenarios needs almost no motivation or willpower to achieve. But, each of them is an excellent step.

Here's how: Decide that your small goal is the minimumyou can achieve, and you'll be able to do more if you're enough.

Most times you'll accomplish better and feel fantastic because you're exceeding your goals. On rare occasions, you'll do only the minimum and be feeling great, as you've accomplished your goals.

How do these small-scale objectives actually have an impact? The reason is that massive change takes tiny steps, which are repeated every day that create momentum and produce positive outcomes over time.

The top 8% of those who succeed know this, yet the majority of people don't even try this method because they believe it's useless to start with something so small. Wrong! As time passes, hitting your smaller goals will create new habits of mind that will lead you towards rewiring your mind to allow you to achieve your greatest goals.

7. Make yourself familiar in getting comfortable with the "F" word - The steps to alter your attitude that I've laid out so far will enable you to take the next step with confidence towards realizing more of your goals and desires. But, it's important to recognize that this will take a lot of effort.

This is why the most successful people like the F word FAILURE.

When people hit an obstacle, they create excuses or quit. The most successful people recognize they are the sole thing which can hinder them from achieving their goals is not doing... therefore they do not! They are aware that they encounter difficulties and may even fail on the journey.

Conclusion

Your brain can be adapted. It is possible to rewire your brain to think and perform actions that can improve your life in all aspects in your daily life and and especially the future. This idea actually offers two benefits, as it is believed that the Law of Attraction states that you are what you believe about. This means that not only can change your brain's wiring to make sure that your default setting can be positive but by doing so, you'll also utilize your Law of Attraction. The way you feel will no longer dictate how you feel, but instead you'll be able to master your emotions. You'll learn to communicate with your emotions how you feel and, with time it will be an habit that you can be proud of.

www.ingramcontent.com/pod-product-compliance
Lightning Source LLC
Chambersburg PA
CBHW060333030426
42336CB00011B/1327